HOSPITAL
SMARTS

HOSPITAL
SMARTS

The Insider's Survival Guide to

Your Hospital, Your Doctor, the Nursing Staff—

and Your Bill!

Theodore Tyberg, M.D., and Kenneth Rothaus, M.D.

HEARST BOOKS

NEW YORK

To Paula and Tara

Library of Congress Cataloging-in-Publication Data

Tyberg, Theodore.
    Hospital smarts : the insider's survival guide to
your hospital, your doctor, the nursing staff—and your bill! /
    Theodore Tyberg and Kenneth Rothaus.
      p. cm.
    Includes index.
    ISBN 0–688–13379–7
    1. Hospital patients. 2. Hospital care. 3. Consumer education.
I. Rothaus, Kenneth. II. Title.
RA965.6.T94 1995
362.1'1—dc20   95–16933
                                     CIP

Printed in the United States of America

First Edition

1 2 3 4 5 6 7 8 9 10

BOOK DESIGN BY LAUREN DONG

ACKNOWLEDGMENTS

This book was written for our patients and their families. Our desire was to give them a better understanding of the hospital environment and in so doing, reduce their fear and anxiety.

The book is dedicated to our families, our wives, our children, and our parents, who put up with our absence on many evenings and weekends while we were writing and rewriting the book. Their support was always there even when we weren't.

Our agent, Sherry Arden Bellak, believed in this book, fought for it, and guided us through the long and sometimes frustrating process. Our editor, Megan Newman, had a vision of what this book should be and molded it for the better over our sometimes strenuous opposition. Special thanks go to Betty Rothbart, M.S.W., a free-lance writer/editor, who assisted us with writing, organizing, and editing the book. When we got lost in the jungle of medical jargon, she guided us back to a path that patients can understand.

We thank the many professionals at the hospital and in our offices who gave advice and information. Jodi Silverman, a dedicated social worker, deserves special mention for the wealth of invaluable information she provided.

CONTENTS

Contents

INTRODUCTION

Each year, thirty-three million people* are admitted to hospitals in the United States. When you are one of them, your happiest moment is usually the day you are discharged. If all has gone well, you are better than when you arrived—and relieved to be returning home. Although hospitalization is sometimes necessary, it is not always pleasant. Life as a patient can be unnerving and intimidating. Hospital admission may entail yielding some control over your body. Medical professionals whom you may have just met touch, prod, and poke areas that have heretofore remained private. Doctors and nurses openly discuss your bodily functions, and while they may be speaking English, their words may be unintelligible jargon.

Hospitals have their own unique customs, language, hierarchy, and pitfalls. Doctors, nurses, and other professionals try to prepare patients for what to expect, but there is not enough time in a day to cover everything. So we have written this book to "translate" hospital life for patients and their families, beginning with the moment you are told that you need admission to the hospital, and ending with post-hospital care at home. Our goal is to explain, warn, prepare, and direct you through a typical hospitalization.

This does *not* mean that we want you to enter the hospital distrust-

---

* American Hospital Association, 1993

ing everything and everybody; that sort of attitude is tension-producing for you, unnecessary, and counterproductive. Patients who are suspicious or overbearing do not receive better care; in fact, some professionals in the hospital even tend to avoid them. Rather, our goal is to help you understand how hospitals function and what questions to ask.

We believe that the best doctor-patient relationship is a partnership, not a dictatorship, and the best conversations are not monologues by either patient or physician, but dialogues that indicate mutual respect. The best doctors *want* their patients to be informed, and the most satisfied patients are those who are as relaxed, confident, and knowledgeable as possible. By demystifying hospital life, we hope to enhance your overall hospital experience.

So use this book as a reference, a guide, or even a pillow, but especially as a tool that can help you to enter and leave the hospital with your health and dignity intact.

CHAPTER 1

GETTING THE NEWS: YOU NEED HOSPITAL CARE

You may be shocked to be told that you need to be hospitalized. The news may seem like a bad dream come true, and so alarm you that logical thought is difficult. On the other hand, you may have suspected that you would need to be hospitalized, and feel relieved to have your feelings confirmed. You may even be looking forward to your hospital stay, as you anticipate getting your medical problem resolved and your life back on track.

In any case, it's usually helpful to have a relative or friend accompany you to your physician's office—to lend moral support, to take notes, and later, to help you recall what the doctor said.

Always go in with a list of questions. Otherwise, you may be too distracted, emotional, or concerned about taking up too much of your doctor's time to remember everything you wanted to talk about. The list of questions will focus your attention and ensure that you will get the information you need.

Do I really need to be in the hospital?

A great many procedures that once required overnight hospitalization are now performed on an outpatient basis: You arrive at the hospital in the morning, have the test, medical treatment, or surgical procedure, and are scheduled to go home the same day, with no overnight stay. (For an explanation of the differences among traditional, outpatient, and same-day admissions, see Chapter 4, "Planning and Preparing for Surgery.")

Because outpatient care is much cheaper than in-hospital care, it is sure to become ever more prevalent as health insurers and the government attempt to reduce medical costs. The trend is to shift any procedure that can be done without staying in a hospital bed overnight to an outpatient setting. For example, people were once routinely hospitalized for cardiac catheterization, which is now just as routinely done on an outpatient basis.

Whether you really need to be hospitalized hinges on how sick your physician judges you to be. It's important that you understand how serious your medical problem is, what your alternatives are, and the potential consequences of *not* being hospitalized.

You have the final say in any planned treatment, including hospitalization. Make sure your doctor describes your treatment plan in jargon-free language, and explains why it must be done in the hospital. Your doctor will probably have to explain the proposed treatment plan to your insurer as well, to justify the projected expense.

What kind of hospital will I go to?

Many doctors have admitting privileges at several hospitals, and some hospitals have greater expertise in certain medical problems. For example, diagnostic workups and such relatively simple procedures as cardiac catheterization can almost always be handled safely and effectively in a community (nonuniversity-associated) hospital. However, a balloon angioplasty, which is a more complex procedure with greater potential risks, requires the on-site backup of a cardiac surgery team, something a community hospital may lack.

How long will I have to be in the hospital?

Physicians used to be able to answer this question by themselves. But in today's cost-cutting climate, your insurance company frequently dictates the length of your hospitalization. For many nonemergency admissions, insurance companies devise a formula determining how many days of hospitalization they are willing to pay for. For example, a patient admitted for an appendectomy may be allotted three days. If complications arise, requiring prolonged hospitalization, the doctor must contact the insurance company, explain the situation, and receive permission for the patient to stay longer.

Such permission is not always granted. Insurance companies would rather pay less than more, so sometimes they insist that a patient go home before either the patient, family, or physician feels ready. (For further discussion of hospital costs, see Chapter 5, "Dollars and Sense.")

Who will be in charge of my care?

The doctor who arranges your admission is usually the one in charge while you are in the hospital. In some instances, however, a physician may arrange to have you admitted under a different specialist's care. For example, if you need abdominal surgery, your internist may have a general surgeon admit you to a surgical floor. The doctor in charge will oversee the orders the nursing staff receives for your care, as well as the interns, residents, and fellows assigned to you during your hospitalization.

Will I be in the hospital over the weekend?

You probably don't want to be admitted on a Friday for a series of tests, since you might be lying around over the weekend with nothing going on. Most doctors work a five- or six-day week and arrange for other doctors to cover their patients over weekends and holidays. A covering doctor answers phone calls, makes hospital rounds, and generally assumes responsibility in the absence of the "covered doctor." But covering doctors generally do not know the patients as well as the primary physician, so they are often reluctant to do anything other

---

AFTER YOUR HOSPITAL STAY

You will need recuperation time when you go home from the hospital. Ask your doctor what to expect, plan accordingly, and don't be too ambitious about rushing back into your normal routine.

CHECKLIST FOR MAKING ARRANGEMENTS

Before entering the hospital, here are some things you may need to do:

☐ **Arrange child care, car pools, and school-related matters.**

☐ **Plan for pet and plant care, grocery shopping, cooking, snow shoveling, and other household responsibilities.**

☐ **Obtain medications, dressings, equipment, or special foods that your doctor recommends.**

☐ **Determine who will handle your responsibilities at work.**

☐ **Arrange storage for your car.**

☐ **Cancel newspaper delivery.**

☐ **Have the post office or a neighbor hold your mail.**

☐ **Give a neighbor or building superintendent the key to your home or the phone number of a friend or relative to call in case of emergency.**

☐ **Arrange for someone to visit or check on your elderly parent(s).**

☐ **Plan for posthospital companionship and care.**

☐ **Plan for adapting your home if you will be disabled (e.g., add a ramp for wheelchair access, install handrails in the tub for balance).**

than maintain the status quo. Only in extreme emergencies do most covering physicians undertake new tests or therapies.

In an emergency situation, of course, you have no choice as to day of admission, and weekend emergency care is almost the same as emergency care during the week.

Should I go into the hospital for an elective procedure in July?

Every July 1, all the interns and residents in the hospital move up a notch in their training, and newly graduated medical students become the new interns. These young doctors are tremendously enthusiastic and eager to please, flush with knowledge gained in four hard years of medical school. If they have arrived from a different hospital, they may need some time to become comfortable with the nuances of that particular hospital, so they may not function as efficiently for the first couple of months as they will once they know their way around. Although some people may feel that going into a hospital in July is like buying a car built on a Monday, if you have to be admitted during that time, do not fear. There are still plenty of medical staff members in the hospital who do know all the ropes: the more senior and the chief residents and, of course, the captain of the ship for your admission: your attending internist or surgeon.

How will I know when to arrive and where to go?

Most hospitals call patients on the day of admission to confirm that a bed is available. Hospital administrators are eager to have as many hospital beds filled as possible, but because patients sometimes don't go home exactly as planned, a bed for a scheduled elective admission isn't always available. So wait until you are called before leaving your home. You can also try calling the admitting office yourself.

Most hospitals like inpatients to arrive at about three o'clock in the afternoon. Patients being discharged have left and housekeeping has had a chance to clean up the room. But don't arrive too late, i.e., after seven o'clock in the evening. Admission testing (usually an EKG, chest X ray, and blood tests) is most efficiently done in the early afternoon. Late arrivals may find themselves sitting in a wheelchair outside an X-ray department, waiting to be squeezed into the emergency schedule for a routine chest X ray.

Outpatient and same-day-admit patients are usually asked to arrive early in the morning.

What should I take to the hospital?

Nightgown or pajamas. You may wish to take your own nightclothes, since hospital gowns are often tattered, missing buttons or snaps, and difficult to tie in a way that adequately covers you, unless you have an advanced degree in mechanical engineering. (The solution: Wear *two* hospital gowns, one tied in the front, the other tied in the back; the overlap gives you full coverage.)

However, you may not wish to wear your own nightclothes all of the time, especially if they are not easy to open. Hospital gowns are easy to manipulate and allow rapid access to your veins for blood drawing as well as to your front and back for examination. And neither you nor anyone else will be upset if the gowns become soiled.

You might be able to wear a sweatsuit or gym shorts if you are near the end of your hospital stay and will not need extensive testing, blood drawing, or frequent examinations.

Bathrobe and slippers. Hospitals tend to be cool (some would say chilly), especially in radiology areas where equipment must be kept cool to work correctly. A robe covers your hospital gown or night-clothes and keeps you from freezing if you are left in the hallway waiting for a test. Slippers will be more comfortable than shoes when you walk to the bathroom or through the corridors.

Entertainment. A hospital stay can be boring. On days when little testing is being done and you feel relatively healthy and alert, you can use the time to read books or magazines, catch up on letter writing, sketch, play solitaire, or do crossword puzzles, needlepoint, or em-broidery. You might like to have a deck of cards or travel-size games of Scrabble, checkers, or backgammon to play with visitors.

Some hospitals offer VCRs and a selection of movies, and every hospital will supply you with a television, often with a built-in radio, for an extra charge.

Medication. Always bring every medication you take routinely, as well as a list of your medications, including oral contraceptives and vitamins or other supplements. The nurses and doctors must know exactly what you are taking and how often. Writing out your medi-cation schedule is immeasurably helpful to the staff and safer for you, and helps avoid needless mistakes.

Pillow. Hospital pillows are covered in plastic to keep them dry and germ-free, but you may find that they are uncomfortable or have an unappealing odor. Though you might be tempted to bring along your own fluffy down pillow, it's better to buy a cheap but comfortable pillow that you won't miss too much if it gets lost or soiled.

Toiletries. Bring a toothbrush, toothpaste, soap, washcloth, comb and brush, deodorant, tampons or sanitary napkins, cosmetics, a small hand mirror, shampoo, and other grooming items.

Notebook and pens. Write down questions for your doctors and nurses in the notebook. Some people also like to jot down test results, thoughts, and feelings, and a list of get-well cards, flowers, gifts, and visitors to acknowledge later.

Phone numbers. You may not want to bring your entire address book to the hospital, but do have with you the phone numbers of people you may want to call from your hospital room. Many hospitals will charge a phone rental fee, even for incoming calls only.

Alarm clock or watch. Bring an inexpensive, lighted alarm clock or watch to the hospital. It will help you get oriented when you awaken (or are awakened), keep track of your medication schedule, and let you know when to expect meals, visitors, and tests.

LEAVE YOUR VALUABLES AT HOME

Resist the temptation to bring expensive things with you, such as computer games and radios, down pillows or comforters, jewelry, or even stylish robes. Valuables unfortunately have a way of disappearing from hospital rooms, and the loss of a favorite item might be hard to bear.

If your admission is an emergency, send your valuables home with your family, or have them catalogued by the nursing staff and placed in the hospital safe for collection when you go home. Don't forget to pick them up on the way out, since it can be a hassle to get them later.

PACKING CHECKLIST

- ☐ nightgown/pajamas
- ☐ robe
- ☐ slippers
- ☐ alarm clock or watch
- ☐ books, magazines
- ☐ stationery, envelopes, stamps
- ☐ address book or list of phone numbers and addresses
- ☐ notebook
- ☐ pens
- ☐ playing cards, games, etc.
- ☐ medication
- ☐ list of medication, schedule, dosages
- ☐ pillow
- ☐ toothbrush
- ☐ toothpaste
- ☐ soap
- ☐ washcloth
- ☐ comb and brush
- ☐ razor and shaving foam
- ☐ small mirror
- ☐ deodorant
- ☐ tampons/sanitary napkins
- ☐ cosmetics
- ☐ other toiletry items
- ☐ other

_____

_____

_____

_____

_____

_____

_____

_____

QUESTIONS FOR YOUR DOCTOR

Do I really need to be in the hospital?

What kind of hospital will I go to?

How long will I have to be in the hospital?

Who will be in charge of my care?

Will I be in the hospital over the weekend?

Should I go into the hospital for an elective procedure in July?

How will I know when to arrive and where to go?

What should I take to the hospital?

Notes:

CHAPTER 2

TYPES OF HOSPITALS

O nce you and your physician have decided that you need to enter a hospital, the next issue is: Which hospital? In some instances, you may not have a choice. For example, if you belong to a health maintenance organization (HMO), you may be limited to hospitals with which your HMO has a contract. (See Chapter 5, "Dollars and Sense.")

However, many private physicians can admit patients to more than one hospital, and will include you in the decision-making process. In order to make an educated choice, it is important to understand the similarities and differences among the three main types of hospitals: teaching hospitals, community hospitals, and Veterans Administration (V.A.) hospitals.

TEACHING HOSPITALS

A teaching hospital is typically affiliated with a university medical school and features a complete staff of senior physicians and eager house staff (see Chapter 14, "Your Hospital Team"). The attending physicians are appointed as professors in the medical school and expected not only to care for patients, but to teach medical students and residents and in many cases to do scientific research as well. These hospitals attract the top graduates of senior medical school classes and are the most prestigious places to practice medicine. Many of the great leaps of medical development have originated in university-affiliated hospitals.

Inner-city hospitals were originally placed in crowded, poor neighborhoods where most of the population did not have a private physician. The inner-city hospitals afforded this poorer population access to quality health care. Some of this country's most famous hospitals, such as Bellevue in New York, are inner-city hospitals. The trade-off for the patients for providing experience to train younger physicians and surgeons was that many stayed on and provided care to the local residents for their entire career.

Hospital structure has changed over the past fifteen years. While the house staff (interns, residents, and fellows) are still responsible for the minute-to-minute patient care, there is far more supervision by senior physicians. There has been a revolution in house-staff hours, responsibility, and supervision. For example, every patient admitted to a hospital in New York must have an identifiable attending physician responsible for his or her care. House staff (also called house officers) must no longer work the crushing hours of yesteryear and must be sent home after twenty-four straight hours of work.

COMMUNITY HOSPITALS

Community hospitals (sometimes called suburban hospitals) are a by-product of the migration of people out of the cities and into ever-growing suburban areas. As areas become more populous, a hospital is needed, and since it's rarely possible to modify an existing building, the hospital is newly built. Therefore, community hospitals are generally newer and more attractive than inner-city teaching hospitals, and often feature more adequate parking and security, although it is just as necessary in community as in other types of hospitals to take safety precautions.

Even the food at community hospitals tends to be better, and the price of a room is almost always lower. Since many suburban areas are relatively affluent, patients generally have insurance to pay their bills; because the hospital does not have to absorb the bills of people who cannot pay, have no insurance, or have poverty-related illnesses, hospitals can charge less.

The nursing staff in these hospitals tends to have lower job turnover. Perhaps nurses stay in their jobs longer because they function more independently in these hospitals than in teaching hospitals, and the environment may be more pleasing. Since community hospitals have few or no house officers, interns, and residents, the nursing staff fulfills the role of interns and takes orders directly from the attending physicians. If you are sick in the middle of the night, the nursing staff holds the fort until the attending staff arrives.

Medical and surgical procedures are performed by attending physicians, not by interns or medical students. Thirty years ago, care at these community hospitals tended to be provided primarily by general practitioners; specialty care (e.g., cardiologic care) required transfer to a teaching hospital. Nowadays, specialists and subspecialists have become so numerous that even the smallest hospitals are staffed by excellent subspecialty physicians. Transfer to university hospitals is now required mainly for certain complex procedures that entail high costs for equipment and personnel that cannot be supported by a small number of patients.

Occasionally, medical colleges associate themselves with outlying community hospitals, thus giving them the cachet of a university center. While this does not guarantee quality, university-associated community hospitals must adhere to quality-of-care criteria established by the parent institution, and the medical staff must fulfill the credentialing criteria necessary for a medical school appointment.

VETERANS ADMINISTRATION HOSPITALS

Veterans Administration (V.A.) hospitals provide free care to a specific clientele: past or present members of the armed forces of the United States, and their dependents. These hospitals offer the same medical services as most university hospitals and are frequently associated with schools of medicine. House-staff members from associated teaching hospitals often do stints at the V.A.

V.A. hospitals are especially recognized for their care of patients with chronic disease (such as severe chronic bronchitis or complications of diabetes), and for their rehabilitation of patients with catastrophic injuries, such as those sustained in combat or auto accidents. Another example of where Veterans Administration hospitals excel is in treatment of patients who have had an amputation.

■   ■   ■

So if you happen to have a choice, which type of hospital should you choose? The quality of physician care has become more uniform at these different hospitals, but the availability of specific tests, operations, or subspecialists may differ. Chronic illnesses that require long-term care, such as the rehabilitation phase after a stroke, may be best treated at Veterans Administration hospitals where long-term residence is the norm and the administration is not in a hurry to discharge you. Acute, very complex problems such as severe heart attacks, which require greater specialization, resources, and medical technologies, or rare operations, such as the removal of a pancreatic cancer, are best dealt with at university centers. Elective operations such as face-lifts or diagnostic evaluation such as breast biopsies can be handled quite well at a community hospital with its more pleasant amenities. If you have any doubt about which hospital to choose, ask your doctor how many cases like yours a particular hospital handles in a year.

UNIVERSITY VERSUS COMMUNITY HOSPITALS
Examples of What to Do Where

UNIVERSITY HOSPITAL	COMMUNITY HOSPITAL
Organ transplantation	Treatment of pneumonia
Burn treatment	Abdominal surgery
Pediatric cardiac surgery	Arthroscopy
Massive trauma	Medical workup

TRANSFERS

Occasionally, if you require a test or operation that is not available at a particular hospital, you will be transferred to another institution. Some hospitals have both financial and teaching links and a formal arrangement for patient transfer in place.

A problem may arise if you have an emergency admission to a hospital in which you have never been a patient. Should this occur in New

York State, for reimbursement reasons it is difficult to be transferred to another hospital if the second hospital offers a procedure or test that the first hospital cannot perform.

The conclusion: If you must get sick at all, try to do so near your favorite hospital.

CHAPTER 3

CONSULTATION WITH A SURGEON

L ike most people, you probably consulted an internist or family practitioner for a medical workup at the first sign of a medical problem. And you may have been surprised when the internist determined that you might need surgery or that your problem could be properly diagnosed only by a surgeon. Now you find yourself with a referral to a general surgeon or a surgical specialist, such as a hand surgeon, head-and-neck surgeon, plastic surgeon, gynecologist, pediatric surgeon, or thoracic surgeon. (If you are already hospitalized, the internist arranges for a surgeon to visit your hospital room for an in-patient consultation.) You need to meet with the surgeon, clarify your medical situation, and make some important decisions.

Surgeons, to an even greater degree than internists, are very highly specialized. While cardiologists, gastroenterologists, endocrinologists, and other specialists in internal medicine spend some or most of their day practicing general internal medicine, most surgeons practice only their specialty. Even so-called general surgeons are highly specialized compared to their counterparts of just a few decades ago, who operated on almost any area of the body. Thirty years ago, for example, on a given day, a general surgeon might have operated on a finger tendon, removed a patient's thyroid cancer, performed a hysterectomy, and biopsied a tumor in a patient's lung. Today, those same procedures would be done by surgical specialists: a hand surgeon, head-and-neck surgeon, gynecologist, and thoracic surgeon.

Specialists have proliferated because improved technologies have enabled surgeons to handle more difficult problems with increasing success—and these new procedures require greater knowledge and training. To gain the necessary skills and knowledge, surgeons must spend more and more time in specialized training, and they soon begin to treat these areas exclusively—as their specialty.

Specialty training has greatly benefited patients. Specialists' new expertise, in concert with new technologies, enables them to successfully treat problems that were not correctable before. For example, a pediatric heart surgeon can now treat forms of congenital heart disease that in the past would have been fatal. A hand surgeon can repair and save an injured finger tendon that once would have resulted in a permanent loss of motion. Now the patient can reasonably expect not only to regain the motion of that tendon but to return to work.

You may wish to go directly to a specialist your internist recommends, or to ask for names of two doctors to choose between. Seek a board-certified specialist; you can obtain names or check qualifications by contacting specialty societies, such as the American Society of Plastic and Reconstructive Surgeons.

WHEN PLANNING AN ELECTIVE SURGICAL PROCEDURE

It is crucial to check with your insurance carrier well in advance of the scheduled surgery date. Many carriers require mandatory second opinions or at least preapproval prior to the surgery if your benefits are to be valid. See Chapter 5, "Dollars and Sense."

COMMUNICATING WITH YOUR SURGEON

Whatever your medical problem, the surgeon has to evaluate your entire medical situation to confirm or supply the diagnosis and to outline a treatment plan. The surgeon reads your medical records or hospital chart, speaks to your internist, takes a history, examines you, then recommends a course of treatment or presents alternatives.

But the process of planning your medical treatment doesn't end there. A consultation with a surgeon is a two-way street: You, the patient, must clearly understand the surgeon's findings and recommendations in order to make decisions and to give your informed consent. It is important to ask questions that will help you to do so.

All surgeons expect patients to ask questions; don't hesitate out of concern that you are imposing on the doctor's time. Answering your questions is just as much a part of the surgeon's job as reading an X ray or using a scalpel. At the same time, some doctors are better than others at communicating. You may have to remind the doctor to speak in plain English, for example, rather than in medical jargon. Some doctors tend to skimp on details, often out of concern that certain information may unnecessarily alarm or confuse the patient. If you want more in-depth information, say so.

At the same time, you need to be sensitive to how much information is "too much." It is not always appropriate to expect a surgeon to describe at great length highly complex technical procedures that took him or her many years of education and training to understand. Furthermore, in this age of litigation, some doctors tend to be leery of patients who ask an overabundance of questions, especially if those patients seem to have a belligerent or challenging attitude. Doctors should never be too busy to answer patients' legitimate questions, even if they are plentiful; but nor should patients expect doctors to spend hours giving them a personal seminar. If the balance seems difficult to achieve, you may try writing a letter to the doctor listing all the questions, so that he or she can have a chance to organize a response. You might also want to ask if the doctor has handouts or can recommend articles that describe a particular treatment or procedure. But if the communication between you and a surgeon is truly difficult, seek another doctor with whom you have better chemistry and a better chance to get the information and rapport you need.

Following are questions for the surgeon that can help you understand your situation and make decisions.

What is the problem?

Make sure you understand exactly what the surgeon believes is wrong. If the doctor uses medical terms that you don't understand, request an explanation in "plain English." It is often helpful to ask the doctor to show you the site of your problem in an anatomy book or on an anatomical model, or to do a quick sketch.

You also have the right to see and request explanations of your X rays and other test results. The better you are able to visualize the situation, the more competent you will be in making a decision on how to proceed.

What method or surgical procedure do you recommend for treating and correcting the problem? Why do you believe this is the best approach?

Make sure you understand what the treatment involves, as well as what follow-up care will be needed.

What alternative procedures—including not having surgery—are available?

You always have choices. Surgeons may differ in what they think may be the best approach for a particular problem. For example, one surgeon may recommend a lumpectomy with radiation for a woman with breast cancer, while another may suggest a mastectomy. One surgeon may recommend radiation as a treatment for prostate cancer, while another favors surgery. All of these surgeons have data to support their position. Knowing the alternatives—and noticing which of these your surgeon recommends—educates you about the problem. If you are unsure or unhappy with a surgeon's approach, seek a second opinion.

Explore the option of having no surgery at all. What are the consequences—in terms of quality of life, general health, prognosis, and life expectancy—if you decide to leave a problem alone? What are the statistics? Can you delay surgery? How fast might the situation worsen? Or is it likely to stay the same for a while—and if so, for how long? Are there nonsurgical treatments that could help you delay or avoid surgery?

What are the expected results?

Surgery does not always cure a problem; it may ameliorate but not eliminate it. You may or may not be able to resume your normal activities—either immediately, or months later, or ever. Make sure your doctor is very clear about what you can expect. Will heart surgery enable you to resume exercising? When? Will surgery on your knee restore your full range of motion? Will surgery on or near your reproductive organs affect your fertility?

What are the potential risks and complications?

All surgery involves risks. Surgery might not be successful. You could have an adverse reaction to certain types of anesthesia. There are risks of infection or bleeding, or other nearby structures may be damaged.

Yet there are also risks associated with *not* doing surgery. The decision to proceed is based on a belief that the benefits of surgery significantly outweigh the risks.

What type of anesthesia is required? Is there a choice of general or local anesthesia? Do you pick the anesthesiologist or work with the same group of anesthesiologists all the time?

Different types of anesthesia present their own benefits and risks, and certain anesthesiologists are more skilled or experienced than others. Ask your surgeon what your options are. See Chapter 16, "Anesthesia and Pain Management."

What happens if something unexpected, such as a tumor, is discovered during surgery?

With all the excellent diagnostic tools such as CAT Scan and MRI (see Glossary of Procedures) that are available today, your surgeon should have a pretty clear idea of what the possibilities are and discuss them with you prior to surgery. Surprises are highly unusual. If surgeons discover a condition that is life-threatening and requires immediate action, they are obligated to proceed. In a less critical situation, they seek immediate consultation with the family or wait until the patient is awake and has left the recovery room.

How long will the operation take, and how long will I be in the recovery room?

Your family will appreciate a "ballpark" estimate of how long the operation will take—and, therefore, how long they will have to wait before receiving word from your surgeon that all went well. Recovery-room time is generally one to two times the duration of the anesthesia (see Chapter 18, "The Recovery Room").

Will I require a blood transfusion?

Certain types of surgery, such as most abdominal hernia repairs, very rarely require blood transfusions; in other types, transfusions are more common. If your surgeon advises that a transfusion might be necessary, you may wish to explore the possibility of donating your own blood in advance (autotransfusion) or having your family donate blood (directed donation). For a discussion of blood transfusion possibilities, see Chapter 4, "Planning and Preparing for Surgery."

How much postsurgical pain will I have and how long will my recuperation take?

If you are considering surgery for a nonemergency condition, the answer to this question will help you plan the best time to schedule the operation. For example, if you are a dedicated teacher who wants to miss as few work days as possible, you may decide to schedule surgery at the beginning of your summer vacation.

Where will my incision be and what will it look like?

In some instances, you can "negotiate" with your surgeon about an incision's size or location. For example, a woman who needs a cesarean-section delivery or surgery to remove an ovarian cyst might wish to request a low, horizontal "bikini cut" incision that would not show when she wears a bikini, instead of a vertical incision that she might want to cover with a one-piece bathing suit. Models, actors, and other people who want to avoid conspicuous scars should share their concerns with their surgeons. Sometimes a technique might be used that minimizes scarring, or your surgeon might recommend a consultation with a plastic surgeon for postsurgical planning. Many women who are having an elective cesarean section arrange to have a plastic surgeon close their incision. In most cases, this is not covered by health insurance.

How complicated a bandage or dressing will I have to change? When will my stitches come out?

The answer to this question will indicate whether you will need a relative or home-care worker to provide assistance after surgery, or whether you will be able to handle your bandage yourself.

When can I resume normal activities?

Again, the answer will help you decide when the best time is to schedule surgery. People are often concerned about how soon they can do the following things.

Lift, care for, and play with children. A parent's surgery can be a mystifying and distressing event for children, especially babies and very young children who must be deprived of breast, cuddling, and the parent's presence for a day or more. A woman who does not want to interrupt breastfeeding may decide to postpone elective surgery for several months. A man who coaches his daughter's Little League base-ball team may want to postpone his surgery until after the team's "World Series" playoffs—and then enjoy a leisurely recuperation while his daughter is away at camp.

Exercise. If your regular exercise must be curtailed, explore with your surgeon what alternative forms of exercise you might try. For example, if you are a runner who needs knee surgery, you might be able to swim sooner than you can resume running. You might also be able to use weights to maintain upper-body strength while your leg heals.

If you have led a sedentary lifestyle but would like to begin exercising, ask your surgeon for guidance as to appropriate types of exercise, and the pace at which you should progress once you get the doctor's go-ahead to proceed.

Return to work. If you must lose time from work, will you be able to do any paperwork or computer work while recuperating?

Have sex. The answer to this question, of course, affects both patient and partner. Both should know in advance how long they must abstain from sexual activities.

Return to a normal diet or weight loss/gain diet. Surgery may require dietary restrictions, sometimes for only a day or so before surgery, sometimes for a more extended period of time.

Shower. Bathing, hygiene, and other aspects of self-care are important to people of all ages. Knowing in advance the extent of discomfort and inconvenience one can expect is invaluable in helping a person schedule self-care.

Take regular medication, vitamins, or other supplements. Certain medications, etc., must be suspended before, during, and/or after surgery. (See Chapter 4, "Planning and Preparing for Surgery.")

What postoperative doctor visits or other postoperative care will I require?

Postoperative procedures range from a single visit to the surgeon after surgery to an extensive program of physical therapy, rehabilitation, chemotherapy, radiation, or other measures.

MAKING A DECISION

Once your surgeon answers all of these questions to your satisfaction, you can make an informed decision, or decide to get a second, or even a third, opinion first.

If you choose to proceed with surgery, you must sign an informed-consent form. This is a contract between you and the surgeon and the hospital where your procedure will be performed. By signing this contract, you are stating that you understand what will be done, that you have discussed all the indications and complications with the surgeon, and that you are giving your permission to proceed. The one difference between this contract and any other you may have ever signed is that it is not negotiable. None of the printed words can be changed. On the other hand, you have the right to withdraw your consent up until the last minute (see page 32).

The surgeon is limited to performing the procedure as listed on the form. For example, if the listed procedure is removal of a gallbladder, the surgeon does not have the authority to take a skin tag off your big toe after you have been sedated or anesthetized. However, in the unusual event that a potentially life-threatening condition such as a stomach tumor is discovered during surgery and no family member is available for consent, the doctor should proceed with whatever is best for your medical care.

If you will have a same-day admission (see Chapter 4, "Planning and Preparing for Surgery"), once you have signed the informed-consent form, the surgeon's staff will make an appointment for you to go to the office or the hospital the week before surgery for a preoperative history, physical examination, laboratory tests and X rays, and completion of health insurance forms (see Chapter 5, "Dollars and Sense").

Ask your surgeon for written preoperative instructions, for there is much you must know in order to prepare for your operation.

PREOPERATIVE ADULT MEDICAL QUESTIONNAIRE

NAME: _____

AGE: _____ WEIGHT: _____ HEIGHT: _____ BIRTH DATE: _____

ADDRESS: _____ PHONE: (___) ___ - _____

_____ ZIP CODE: _____

I. GENERAL:
(Check One)

YES	NO		
☐	☐	1)	Are you in overall good health?
☐	☐	2)	In the last 6 months have you lost more than 5 lbs?
☐	☐	3)	Do you vomit after eating or drinking?
☐	☐	4)	Have you or any relative had problems with anesthesia?
			If yes, please describe: _____
			_____
☐	☐	5)	Do you live alone?
☐	☐	6)	Do you need help caring for yourself?
		7)	When was your last complete physical? _____ (Date)
☐	☐	8)	Do you have fainting spells?
☐	☐	9)	Do you have epilepsy or seizures?
☐	☐	10)	Do you have, or have you had, cancer?
☐	☐	11)	Have you been treated for cancer? If yes, by what method (e.g., radiation, chemotherapy, etc.): _____

II. HEART:

YES	NO		
☐	☐	1)	Do you have heart disease?
☐	☐	2)	Do you have high blood pressure?
☐	☐	3)	Have you ever had a "heart attack"? When? _____
☐	☐	4)	Do you have chest pain? How often? _____
			What produces it? _____
☐	☐	5)	Have you ever had rheumatic fever?
☐	☐	6)	Have you ever been told you have a heart murmur?
☐	☐	7)	Do you have mitral valve prolapse?
☐	☐	8)	Have you been told to take antibiotics before surgery or dental work?
☐	☐	9)	Do you have an irregular pulse or heart beat?
☐	☐	10)	Have you ever been in heart failure?

III. RESPIRATORY:

YES NO

☐ ☐ 1) Do you have a breathing problem?

☐ ☐ 2) Do you have a cold, running nose, sore throat, or flu?

☐ ☐ 3) Do you have a cough? For how many weeks have you had it?

☐ ☐ 4) Do you bring up anything with the cough?

☐ ☐ 5) Do you smoke? How many packs/day? _____

             For how many years? _____

             6) How many stairs can you climb without getting short of breath? _____

             7) How many blocks can you walk without shortness of breath? _____

☐ ☐ 8) Do you have hay fever?

☐ ☐ 9) Do you have asthma?

☐ ☐ 10) Have you been treated in an emergency room for asthma?

☐ ☐ 11) Have you been treated with steroids?

             12) Name, dosage, and date of last steroid. _____

☐ ☐ 13) Do you have, or have you had, Tuberculosis?

☐ ☐ 14) Have you been exposed to a person with tuberculosis?

☐ ☐ 15) Do you have night sweats? If yes, please explain:

             _____

IV. G.I.:

YES NO

☐ ☐ 1) Do you have loose teeth, dentures, bridge work, or caps?

☐ ☐ 2) Do you have a hiatus hernia?

☐ ☐ 3) Do you have esophagitis or food regurgitation?

☐ ☐ 4) Have you ever had jaundice or hepatitis?

             White type? _____

             When? _____

V. ENDOCRINE:

YES NO

☐ ☐ 1) Are you a diabetic?

☐ ☐ 2) Do you take insulin?

☐ ☐ 3) Do you take oral antihypoglycemics?

☐ ☐ 4) Do you take thyroid medication?

☐ ☐ 5) Do you take steroids (cortisone)?

VI. OBSTETRICS:

YES NO

☐ ☐ 1) Are you or do you believe you could be pregnant?

             2) Date of last menstrual period? _____

VII. TRANSFUSION:

YES   NO

☐   ☐   1) Have you ever had a blood transfusion?

☐   ☐   2) Have you had a blood transfusion within the last 3 months?

☐   ☐   3) Have you ever had a reaction or an allergy to a blood transfusion?

☐   ☐   4) Have you ever been told that you have antibodies against red blood corpuscles or red cells?

☐   ☐   5) Have you been pregnant at any time within the last 3 months?

☐   ☐   6) Have you ever given birth to a baby that had severe yellow jaundice or needed a blood transfusion soon after birth?

☐   ☐   7) Have you been told that you had "Rh Disease"?

☐   ☐   8) Have you or any relative had a bleeding problem, or easy bruising?

☐   ☐   9) Have you donated autologous (your own) or directed (your family or friends) donor blood for own use?*

*(A POSITIVE RESPONSE REQUIRES THAT THE BLOOD BANK RECEIVES A REQUEST FOR BLOOD AND HAS A CURRENT SPECIMEN)

NOTE: The potential use of blood products and transfusions should be discussed with your surgeon prior to surgery.

VIII. List all drugs, medications, eye drops, etc. that you take (including aspirin, Motrin, and Tylenol):

Drugs	Dose	Times/day	Route (mouth, subcut.)
1)			
2)			
3)			

IX. Do you take any street drugs: marijuana, cocaine, etc.? Which ones? How often?

1) _____

2) _____

X. Have you ever had a drinking problem? Have you had a drink in the last 24 hours?

_____

XI. List all prior operations and approximate dates:

1) _____

2) _____

3) _____

XII. List all drug allergies:

Drugs	Type of reaction
1)	
2)	
3)	

XIII. List all handicaps or physical disabilities, glasses, hearing aid, contact lenses, cane, walker, etc.:

1) _____

2) _____

XIV. List all current conditions: _____

_____

_____

XV. Name and phone of person who will escort you home on day of surgery (this is a mandatory requirement):

Name: _____

Phone: _____

XVI. Name, address, and phone of your primary care physician:

Name: _____

Address: _____

Phone: _____

Please list a phone number where you can be reached during the day if further information is needed: (___) ___ - _____

_____	_____	_____	☐☐☐☐☐	_____
PATIENT SIGNATURE	DATE	PHYSICIAN SIGNATURE	(CODE)	DATE

EXAMPLE OF GENERAL PREOPERATIVE INSTRUCTIONS

JANE DOE, M.D.
734 EAST MAIN STREET
SOMEWHERE, USA 12345
(333) 333–3333

GENERAL OPERATIVE INSTRUCTIONS PRINTED FOR: _____
(PATIENT'S NAME)

DATE OF SURGERY: _____ REVIEWED WITH: _____
(FOR DR. JANE DOE)

PATIENT'S SIGNATURE: _____

No aspirin or Ibuprofen or products containing aspirin, including Motrin, Advil, or other nonsteroidal anti-inflammatory agents for **two** weeks prior to surgery. You may take Tylenol.

Limit alcohol intake **one** week prior to surgery and **one** week following surgery to one glass of wine per day.

Nothing by mouth (food or liquid) after midnight the evening prior to surgery.

Office Surgery Patients: Blood work must be done within **two** weeks prior to surgery. A prescription for blood work will accompany these instructions. You may have your blood drawn at ABC Clinical Laboratory or at Elsewhere General Hospital. We must have written lab results prior to surgery.

Hospital Patients: Blood work will be performed at Elsewhere General within **ten** days of the surgery. You will receive all necessary paperwork from this office during your preoperative appointment.

On the day of surgery, please do not wear any makeup or jewelry to the office or hospital.

Take pain medicine as needed postoperatively. Please fill your prescriptions prior to surgery. **Make sure this office has a list of all medications, vitamins, and health food supplements you are currently taking and alert us to any allergies to medications or latex.**

Hospital and Office Patients: **You must be accompanied home by someone after surgery.** You may **not** leave alone via car service or cab.

Prior to surgery, sun exposure (not burning) is acceptable.

All surgical scars must be protected from the sun for **three** months postoperatively. Use a sunblock with SPF 15 or higher.

Provide your doctor with an up-to-date list of all medications you are taking, and their dosages. This is critically important. Some medications may have to be stopped entirely before surgery; some medications may have to be changed; and you may have to take some medications the morning of surgery with a sip of water or wait until after surgery to resume taking them.

Make sure to include on your list *all* prescription *and* over-the-counter medications, oral contraceptives, vitamins and other nutritional supplements, and any homeopathic, herbal, or other therapeutic substances you take on a regular or occasional basis. Don't make assumptions that supposedly "nonmedicinal" items are OK without checking with your doctor. For example, garlic supplements and vitamin E taken in large doses can cause excessive bleeding.

IF YOU ARE ALLERGIC TO LATEX

Let your surgeon know ahead of time so that latex-free gloves can be special-ordered for your operation. An allergy to latex is rare but can be life-threatening.

Follow your doctor's instructions to avoid medications that inhibit blood clotting. Certain medications, including aspirin and non-steroidal anti-inflammatory drugs (NSAIDs), prevent blood from coagulating, or clotting, and present a significant risk during and after surgery. Therefore, in the two weeks before surgery, avoid taking aspirin, any medication that contains aspirin, or any NSAIDs, such as ibuprofen. To be safe, check with your surgeon before taking *any* medication, vitamin, or other supplement in the two weeks before surgery.

In addition, anticoagulation medication such as Coumadin or Heparin must be stopped prior to any surgical procedure. But stopping is not always simple; it must be done very carefully and only under the doctor's supervision. Some individuals who have taken anticoagulation medications on a long-term basis may not be able to have the medication stopped because of the high risk that they may develop clots in their leg or heart, then throw emboli to the lungs or brain. For these patients, the risk of stopping the medication is greater than any benefit they may derive from the surgical procedure, and the operation is not done.

PERMISSION FOR OPERATION

I hereby give authorization and consent to Dr. _____

and the hospital and its staff to perform an operation described as

_____

_____
(DESCRIBE OPERATION)

upon _____ .
(NAME OF PATIENT)

The nature, intended purpose, and significant risks and consequences of such operation, as well as the alternatives if the operation is not performed, have been explained to and discussed

with me by _____ , and I give this permission with full
(NAME OF PHYSICIAN)

knowledge and understanding thereof. I understand that medicine is not an exact science and the possibility that the operation may not have the benefits or result intended. I am also aware that there are always risks and dangers to life and health associated generally with anesthesia, surgery, use of medication, medical procedures and treatments that can cause adverse consequences not ordinarily anticipated in advance, but I give this permission with full assent nevertheless.

I further grant permission for the use of such tissues and/or organs, as it may be necessary to remove during said operation, for purposes of pathological diagnosis and thereafter for the advancement of medical science and education, and their disposal, at this hospital or at such other institution as this hospital may designate.

*Signature _____

_____
(RELATIONSHIP TO PATIENT)

Date _____

*NOTE: If the patient is under eighteen (18) years, the permission of the patient's parent or legal guardian must be obtained, unless the patient is married or the parent of a child.

I have discussed the nature and purpose of the above operation, and the associated risks, consequences and available alternatives, with the person signing above, and I am satisfied that he/she understands them.

_____M.D.
(SIGNATURE OF PHYSICIAN PROVIDING EXPLANATION)

STERILIZATION REQUEST AND CONSENT

I hereby request the hospital and give authorization to Dr. _____
and the hospital's staff for the sterilization of myself by the following method:

_____
(DESCRIPTION OF PROCEDURE)

I understand the nature of the sterilization procedure described above, the significant medical
risks associated with the procedure (including _____
_____)

and the significant discomforts to be expected as a result of the procedure (including _____
_____)
(TYPE AND APPROXIMATE EXPECTED DURATION OF DISCOMFORTS)

I understand fully that the intended effect of the sterilization requested is to make me permanently incapable of reproducing and having children, and that such a sterilization should be
considered an irreversible procedure.

I am also aware that medicine is not an exact science and that there are always risks and dangers to life and health associated with anesthesia and medical procedures which can cause
adverse consequences not ordinarily anticipated in advance. Furthermore, I am aware that in
rare cases a sterilization does not have the permanency intended and that in such cases the
body may regenerate its reproductive functions.

The matters described in this request and authorization have been explained to and discussed
with me by _____ , and I have been offered
(NAME OF PHYSICIAN)
a satisfactory opportunity to ask all questions I have had with regard thereto.

_____   _____
PHYSICIAN PROVIDING INFORMATION   PATIENT'S SIGNATURE

_____   _____
              WITNESS   SPOUSE'S SIGNATURE

Date _____

NOTE: (a) If non-therapeutic, this procedure may be performed only upon a person competent to give consent to medical treatment under the law of this state, i.e., a person
18 years or older, or any person who has married or is the parent of a child.
  (b) If the patient is married, the consent of the spouse is also required.
  (c) If sterilization is to be performed under any program or project funded, in whole or
part with federal funds, e.g., Medicaid or Medicare, this form <u>AND</u> the additional
special consent form must be completed.

CHAPTER 4

Planning and Preparing
for Surgery

P reparing for surgery is a three-step process: scheduling the operation; taking care of paperwork and other presurgical planning; and having presurgical testing.

SCHEDULING YOUR SURGERY

When to schedule your surgery depends on how urgently you need it. For certain serious medical problems, such as a malignant tumor, obviously, time is of the essence.

But many elective procedures are not associated with life-threatening problems and can be scheduled days, weeks, or even months after your problem is diagnosed. For example, many (though not all) hernia repairs can be put off, as can such procedures as knee arthroscopy (correction of simply injuries to the cartilage and ligaments of the knee). This flexibility enables you to get your affairs in order and choose the most convenient time for both surgery and recuperation.

If your operation requires a long hospitalization or close follow-up, you may want to check if your surgeon has other commitments, such as a medical conference or family vacation, for the week after your

A COMPARISON OF TRADITIONAL, AMBULATORY, AND SAME-DAY ADMISSION SURGERY

Traditional	Ambulatory and Same-Day Admissions
You are admitted at least one night before surgery.	You arrive at hospital morning of surgery.
Blood and urine samples, chest X ray, and cardiogram performed in hospital laboratory following admission.	Testing done as outpatient seven to fourteen days before surgery. (If done sooner than fourteen days, results may no longer be valid. If done closer to the day of surgery than ten days, there may not be enough time to repeat abnormal tests and correct any problems.)
After testing, histories and physical examinations done by attending physician, house staff, nurses, and/or physician's assistant.	Physician does history and physical examinations in advance; nurse (or, in some cases, physician) takes an updated history on morning of surgery.
Any special preparations (e.g., multiple enemas or medications) are ordered and administered by the hospital staff.	You may have to self-administer any special preparations at home before going to hospital.
The evening before surgery, surgeon and anesthesiologist visit your hospital room so you can sign surgical consent forms. Anesthesiologist asks some screening questions.	You sign surgical consent forms in the surgeon's office usually seven to fourteen days before the surgery. You sign the anesthesia consent form during preoperative testing in the hospital or on the day of surgery. Anesthesiologist asks some screening questions.

Traditional	Ambulatory and Same-Day Admissions
Any special diets ordered by surgeon are brought to you by the dietary department; nurses assure that you have nothing to eat or drink after midnight.	You must prepare your own diet and assume responsibility for a complete fast after midnight.
Hospital staff awakens you for early-morning surgery, gives you a hospital gown, and transports you to operating room on a hospital gurney.	You must arrive at hospital very early, e.g., if you have a 7:00 A.M. operation, you must arrive at the hospital at 5:00 A.M. If you live a long distance from the hospital, you may have to spend the night in a nearby hotel in order to be there on time.
After recovery from surgery and anesthesia, you are taken to your hospital room, where you will spend at least one night.	*Ambulatory Admission:* After recovery from surgery and anesthesia, you go home. However, if any complications arise, you may be admitted as an inpatient. *Same-Day Admission:* After recovery from surgery and anesthesia, you are taken to a hospital room, where you will spend at least one night.

procedure. If so, ask who will be covering for your surgeon and decide whether to proceed or to choose an alternate date.

A key consideration in scheduling a surgical procedure is what type of admission it will be. There are three kinds:

Traditional admission. You are admitted to the hospital a day or days before the operation; after surgery, you are taken back to your hospital room and will spend at least one night there.

THE MOST COMMON AMBULATORY PROCEDURES

Service	Procedure	Anesthesia and Approximate Duration
General surgery	Breast biopsy or removal of lump from breast	Local with sedation or general anesthesia (1 hour)
	Inguinal hernia repair	Local with sedation (1 hour)
	Inguinal hernia repair with graft	Local with sedation, regional, or general (2 hours)
Ophthalmology	Cataract removal	Local with sedation (1 hour)
	Repair of detached retina	Local with sedation (2 hours)
Gynecology	D & C (dilatation and curettage)	Regional or general (1/2 hour)
	Pregnancy termination	Regional or general (1/2 hour)
Urology	ESWL (kidney stone removal by sound waves)	Sedation, block, or general (1 hour)
	Cystoscopy	Sedation, block, or general (1 hour)
Plastic and reconstructive surgery	Rhinoseptoplasty ("nose job," repair of deviated or crooked septum)	Local with sedation (1 hour)

Ambulatory admission. You arrive at the hospital the morning of surgery and are discharged after your immediate recovery from the surgery and anesthesia. You are never assigned an inpatient bed; you spend your nonoperative and non–recovery-room time in the ambulatory surgical center.

Same-day admission. You are admitted to the hospital the day of surgery. After the operation, you are taken from the recovery room to an inpatient room, where you will stay at least one night.

In a variation on this theme, some states have a "twenty-three-hour rule." Patients may be admitted to a hospital bed after they leave the recovery room. As long as they are discharged from that bed within twenty-three hours of their original arrival at the admitting office, the procedure is still considered ambulatory, and paid for as such.

PAPERWORK AND PLANNING

Your surgeon's office will guide you through the paperwork that must be completed before surgery, including presurgical, approval, and second-opinion forms required by your health insurance company, Medicaid, or Medicare. Your surgeon's nurse, office manager, or secretary will review all forms and ensure that everything is in order before you enter the hospital. For a discussion of insurance-related paperwork, see Chapter 5, "Dollars and Sense."

But insurance forms are only part of the story. Paperwork and planning also involve taking the following steps.

Read and follow preoperative instructions. Your surgeon will give you verbal or, preferably, written preoperative instructions regarding medications to take or to avoid, dietary restrictions, and other matters. It is crucial to follow these instructions carefully in order to enhance the likelihood that the surgery and recovery will be safe and successful. An example set of preoperative instructions is included in this chapter.

Fill prescriptions for any medications you will need after surgery. Some surgeons prescribe pain medication, antibiotics, and medication for nausea in advance of surgery, so that you have them available immediately.

Fill prescriptions for any special items that have to be ordered and perhaps fitted. For example, you may need special ointments, dressings, garments, braces, or other devices.

Review and sign the surgical consent form. See Chapter 3, "Consultation with a Surgeon," as well as the sample consent form on page 32. Without this "contract" with you, the surgeon cannot proceed.

Arrange to donate blood for your own use if your surgeon recommended autotransfusion. Autotransfusion, also called autologous transfusion, means that you donate your own blood prior to surgery and the blood is held in reserve for you in case you need a transfusion. You usually need to donate the blood at the blood bank within the six weeks prior to surgery, and must follow instructions, take medications if any (such as iron supplements), and sign consent forms. The advantage of donating your own blood is that you do not run the risk of getting hepatitis, HIV, or any other disease from blood donated by someone else.

Some blood banks allow directed transfusions, which use blood donated by individuals chosen by the patient, usually family members. However, just because people are related to you doesn't mean that their blood will be acceptable for your use. Their blood type might not match yours, or they might themselves be infected—perhaps unknowingly—with hepatitis, HIV, or other diseases. Therefore, for your protection, blood banks must screen directed blood just as they screen blood given by any other blood donor. Since blood-bank policies vary state by state, and since even blood banks within the same state may have different internal policies, ask your doctor to check with the blood bank to make sure they screen directed blood. If they do not, have your donors use a blood bank that does.

Follow your doctor's advice about eliminating alcohol before surgery. Most surgeons also ask their patients to avoid any alcohol consumption in the week before surgery. Alcohol can have a deleterious effect on liver function, blood clotting, gastric mucosa, and other body functions.

PRESURGICAL TESTING

Presurgical testing is required for most surgical procedures. Its extent and complexity depend on the proposed surgery and on your age and general health. If you are older than forty, you probably need a full set of blood tests, a urinalysis, an electrocardiogram within the two weeks prior to surgery, and a chest X ray within the last six months, plus a complete history and physical examination. Your surgeon may also require medical clearance by your general practitioner or internist. If you are under forty, you may not be required to have an electrocardiogram or chest X ray.

For certain surgical procedures, such as open-heart surgery or vascular surgery, additional testing may be needed. For example, vascular surgeons have found that a heart attack (myocardial infarction) is the most common cause of significant morbidity (illness or complication) after elective surgery on the aorta and major arteries to the legs. Therefore, they urge all patients to undergo a stress test prior to surgery. The test identifies people who are at high risk for a heart attack. A consulting cardiologist determines whether further testing must be done and what treatments, if any, must be done before, during, and/or after surgery.

Children who are scheduled to have a "routine" procedure, such as a tonsillectomy or repair of an inguinal hernia, are usually only required to have a blood count (hematocrit) and a urinalysis.

TIPS FOR AMBULATORY SURGERY

Since the concept of ambulatory care is relatively recent, how it is handled varies enormously from institution to institution. Hospitals built or extensively remodeled within the last decade have areas dedicated to ambulatory surgery and ambulatory admissions. Older hospitals have had to accommodate ambulatory facilities in an aging physical plant never designed for that purpose. Therefore, an ambulatory patient's experience can range from modern and luxurious to barely tolerable.

You may have to drag your luggage around with you when you arrive at the hospital, and there may not be a secure, guarded area where you can leave your things. Therefore, pack light and only pack things that you won't miss if they disappear. Avoid expensive luggage that could get stolen; use an inexpensive duffel bag or backpack. If you are going to stay overnight and will need more things than can fit in a light bag, arrange for a friend or relative to bring items along later that day, directly to your room.

Even if you are an outpatient, there is always the possibility that you will need to stay overnight; a small percentage of ambulatory patients are admitted because they are excessively sleepy from anesthesia, have too much discomfort, or require intravenous medication or drains. Therefore, plan for a one-night stay and pack accordingly.

Why you have to arrive at the hospital early. When you arrive at the hospital, a clerk reviews your paperwork, then a nurse takes a brief history, makes sure you haven't had anything to eat or drink after midnight, checks your vital signs (temperature, pulse, respiration, and blood pressure), and gives you a hospital gown and perhaps a bag for your clothes and overnight bag. Time elapsed since your arrival: forty-five minutes to an hour. So how come they got you there so early? Contrary to one theory, it's not because the staff had to get there early anyway and did not want to suffer alone!

The answer has to do with operating room schedules and presurgical trouble-shooting. To make the best use of staff members' time and expensive operating room equipment, hospital operating rooms are run on a tight schedule. Hospitals, like airlines, lose money if they "fly empty," so they try not to have any downtime. If the patient who is scheduled before you has canceled, your early arrival enables the hospital to move up the time of your procedure and not lose any operating room time. Early arrival also gives you enough time to straighten out any problems with your paperwork or laboratory results without having to cancel or delay the surgery.

So although it can be aggravating to arrive early only to sit and wait, try to be understanding. Spend the waiting time reading a juicy paperback or flipping through a magazine. Choose inexpensive reading material so you will not be too upset if it ends up misplaced or lost.

PHYSICIAN'S ADMITTING ORDERS

DATE	VALIDATION #

SERVICE
- ☐ MEDICAL SERVICE
- ☐ ORTHOPEDIC SERVICE
- ☐ OPD SERVICE

STATUS
- ☐ EMERGENCY
- ☐ URGENT
- ☐ ELECTIVE
- ☐ SAME-DAY SURGERY
- ☐ AMBULATORY SURGERY

ACCOMMODATIONS
- ☐ ADULT
- ☐ PEDIATRIC
- ☐ ISOLATION
- ☐ PRIVATE
- ☐ SEMI-PRIVATE 2 BEDS
- ☐ SEMI-PRIVATE 4 BEDS

PATIENT'S NAME	SEX ☐ M ☐ F	BIRTH DATE	AGE	HSS#

ADDRESS STREET	CITY	STATE	ZIP CODE

HOME TELEPHONE ( )	OFFICE TELEPHONE ( )	HOSPITAL INSURANCE	☐ COMP AUTHORIZATION ATTACHED

DIAGNOSIS

ADMISSION DATE TIME	☐ NEW ADMISSION ☐ RE-ADMISSION ☐ TRANSFER ☐ UTILIZATION NOTIFIED	CONSULATION WITH

PRE-ADMISSION TESTING	☐ LAB ORDERS _____	☐ ☐ NO. OF UNITS AUTO DESIG
☐ HSS PAT	☐ X-RAY ORDERS _____	DATE/TIME 1 / DATE/TIME 2
☐ OUTSIDE PAT	☐ ADDITIONAL ORDERS _____	DATE/TIME 3
REQUESTED DATE		☐ PHOTO AUTHORIZATION ATTACHED

ADMISSION ORDERS	DIET ☐ REGULAR ☐ OTHER	KNOWN PRECAUTIONS/ALLERGIES

☐ MEDICATION (ORDERS HONORED ONLY WITHIN 10 DAYS OF ADMISSION)

☐ LAB

☐ X-RAY

☐ TYPE & CROSS MATCH   ☐ TYPE & SCREEN ONLY   UNITS RED CELLS

☐ ADDITIONAL ORDERS FOR ADMISSION

SURGERY ORDERS	DATE OF SURGERY	TIME OF SURGERY ☐ AM ☐ PM	LENGTH OF OPERATION (HRS)

OPERATIONS: (NOTE EXACT LOCATION AND PROCEDURE NAME)

PROSTHESIS TYPE

SPECIAL INSTRUMENTS/EQUIPMENT

ANESTHESIA PREFERENCE	☐ EPIDURAL	☐ GENERAL	☐ NERVE BLOCK	☐ LOCAL ONLY	☐ LOCAL/ SEDATION	☐ SPECIAL INSTRUCTIONS

REQUESTS
☐ X-RAY ☐ 2 TEAM ☐ VIDEO ☐ IMAGE INTEN ☐ MICROSCOPE ☐ CELL SAVER ☐ FX TABLE ☐ SPINAL CORD MONITORING ☐ BONE BANK (HSS) ☐ FROZEN SECTION ☐ OTHER PATHOLOGY ____

OTHER SPECIAL REQUESTS

SOCIAL WORK and DISCHARGE PLANNING	ESTIMATED LOSS	ANTICIPATED HOSPITAL CARE PLAN
☐ PRIOR HOME CARE ☐ LIVES ALONE ☐ PSYCHOSOCIAL SUPPORT REQUESTED		☐ HOME - NO ASSISTANCE ☐ NURSING HOME ☐ HOME WITH ASSISTANCE ☐ NEEDS EVALUATION ☐ REHAB

ATTENDING PHYSICIAN SIGNATURE _____ PRINT NAME	RESIDENT PHYSICIAN SIGNATURE _____ PRINT NAME

NOTIFICATION DEPARTMENTS	☐ OPERATING ROOM ☐ MATERIAL MANAGEMENT	☐ BIO-MECHANICS ☐ ADMITTING	☐ ANESTHESIOLOGY ☐ UTILIZATION

AMBULATORY SURGERY CENTER HISTORY AND PHYSICAL

AGE	SEX	B/P	P	R	HEIGHT	WEIGHT

CHIEF COMPLAINT: _____

PRESENT ILLNESS: _____

ALLERGIES ☐ NONE   **CURRENT MEDICATIONS** ☐ NONE

LIST: _____   LIST: _____

_____   _____

_____   _____

_____   _____

PAST HISTORY ☐ NON CONTRIBUTORY _____

_____

_____

_____

FAMILY HISTORY ☐ NON CONTRIBUTORY _____

_____

_____

PHYSICAL EXAMINATION   **ABNORMAL FINDINGS**

NORMAL

☐ INTEGUMENT _____   _____

☐ EYES _____   _____

☐ EARS, NOSE, THROAT _____   _____

☐ HEART _____   _____

☐ LUNGS _____   _____

☐ ABDOMEN _____   _____

SEE ATTACHED MEDICAL CONSULTATION: ☐ _____

SIGNATURE _____ M.D./P.A. DATE: _____

DIAGNOSIS: _____

PROPOSED SURGERY: _____

_____

NO CHANGE IN THE PATIENT'S STATUS HAS OCCURRED SINCE THE ABOVE HISTORY AND PHYSICAL WAS PERFORMED ☐

SIGNATURE _____ M.D. DATE: _____
                 SURGEON

43

CHAPTER 5

DOLLARS AND SENSE

In most hospitals, you are not required to settle the bill before you leave. Hospital administrators are aware that you have just been through a major life trauma, and they try to refrain from adding insult to injury by making you pay for it while you still feel shaken and perhaps in pain. But before long, the day of reckoning arrives, and the extent of your insurance coverage—and your prehospital research—determines just how shocking the bill will be.

The concept of medical insurance really took hold after World War II, and has allowed new technologies and therapies to proliferate in many health care settings. In many cases, your insurance will pay for almost your entire hospitalization, regardless of the total cost. But insurance comes in many guises, and various policies offer widely varying levels of coverage. *It is critical to know exactly what your insurance policy covers before you are admitted to the hospital.*

It is prudent, if you are being admitted electively, to write a letter to your insurance company outlining what is to be done. Be sure to include the CPT (Common Procedural Terminology) codes (see page 82) and your policy number. Your doctor's office will be happy to supply you with the necessary information to be sent, or to assist you with the paperwork, if necessary. Ask the insurance company to agree, in writing, to the proposed treatment. While this sounds simple, unfortunately, some insurance policies are written with so many loop-

WHAT TO INCLUDE IN YOUR PREOPERATIVE LETTER

Patient's name
Name of insured
Group policy number
Patient's policy number
Doctor's name
Proposed procedure
ICD-9 and CPT codes

holes that you may still have problems collecting payment. What to do? Be relentless! If they refuse payment after the fact, write them letters, ask your physician's office to write letters, and call repeatedly. If all this fails, hire an experienced attorney. What if the insurance company refuses to pay before you have a procedure done? You have three choices:

1. Cancel it. It's too expensive to pay for out of your own pocket.

2. Get a second opinion. Perhaps the procedure wasn't necessary in the first place. If the second opinion agrees, fight the insurance company as detailed above.

3. Pay for it yourself—not an infrequent occurrence, especially in cosmetic cases. You can discuss this with your physician and even ask if a discount is possible since you are paying the entire cost yourself.

TYPES OF INSURANCE

TYPES OF INSURANCE

Private Insurance
Government-Sponsored
HMO
Managed Care
Worker's Compensation

In general, all insurance policies pay for basic hospitalization, but there can be profound differences in the choices people have as to provider and hospital; the choices their providers have as to recommending tests, referrals, and hospital stays; and the comprehensiveness of care that patients can expect. Here are descriptions of the most common types of plans.

Private Insurance: Blue Cross, Blue Shield, Major Medical

Most patients who have a private, fee-for-service insurance policy generally have a basic Blue Cross plan that covers their hospitalization. Blue Cross policies frequently have a Blue Shield policy that pays part of the doctor's bill. The balance is then paid by the major-medical company. Some policies do not have a Blue Shield component and the major-medical policy "kicks in" at the first dollar.

Most major-medical policies have both a *deductible* and *coinsurance*. A deductible is a percentage of the first dollars spent, up to a maximum amount, that the insurer requires the patient to pay. As in automobile insurance, the higher the percentage and the greater the amount that the patient must pay, the lower the cost of the insurance.

Coinsurance is a little trickier. Essentially, coinsurance means that your major-medical policy will only cover a percentage of the first charges you receive each year. For example, the policy may state that after your deductible, the insurer will pay for 80 percent of the first $4,000. This means that the insurer will *not* pay for 20 percent, or $800 in this example. It is called coinsurance because if your spouse works and has a separate policy that covers you as well, then you can submit this balance to that insurance carrier.

Some patients have supplemental insurance programs that pick up the coinsurance. If you are not covered by any other insurance plan, then coinsurance effectively increases your deductible. In the above example, therefore, after the first $4,000 in charges, the insurer will pay the entire amount. However, there's a catch: Insurance companies generally pay based on what they consider "usual and customary charges." A problem, of course, is that what insurers think doctors should charge is often less than the actual charges. To avoid burdening you with having to pay the difference, some physicians will accept "assignment," that is, the fee that the insurer has determined is reasonable for a particular service. Some surgeons negotiate their policies regarding assignment on a case-by-case basis. Patients have a little more negotiating power for major procedures that are well reimbursed by the insurance carriers.

Physicians who have elected to become "participating" physicians in Medicare are obliged to accept assignment on all Medicare patients. However, they retain the right to decline assignment on non-Medicare patients.

AN EXAMPLE: HOW A PRIVATE INSURANCE PLAN MIGHT WORK

Ms. Isadore has surgery on her knee. The surgeon's fee is $4,000. Her Blue Cross/Blue Shield plan pays $200, leaving a balance of $3,800. Ms. Isadore's major medical policy has a deductible of $300 and pays 80 percent of the first $5,000 (the coinsurance). Therefore, the major-medical company deducts $300 from the balance of $3,800, leaving a total of $3,500. The company then pays 80 percent of this (the coinsurance), or $2,800. Therefore, out of the original bill, $3,000 ($2,800 + $200) has been paid, leaving a balance of $1,000. If Ms. Isadore is covered by a second major-medical policy or a supplemental policy, she can now submit the $1,000 to that company for payment. The second carrier will not review the claim until the primary carrier has been paid.

Cost of operation $4,000
Blue Shield $200
Balance $3,800
Deductible $300
Coinsurance $0.20 \times (\$3,800 - \$300) = \$700$
Major medical pays $3,800 − (deductible + coinsurance) = $2,800
Total insurance payment $200 + $2,800 = $3,000
Balance of $1,000 represents total of deductible and coinsurance.

GOVERNMENT-SPONSORED INSURANCE PLANS

The main government-sponsored plans are Medicare and Medicaid. Medicare is for people who are elderly (over sixty-five) and disabled (for example, people on kidney dialysis) and is run by the federal government. Medicaid, for people whose incomes and family resources place them below the nationally defined poverty level, is run by the local or state government.

These plans have very specific allowable charges for all medical procedures and professional medical services. Charges for Medicaid tend to be substantially lower than those for Medicare, which in turn are substantially lower than those of private insurance. For example, the fee for an office visit by a Medicaid patient in New York City is $12— regardless of how complex or time-consuming the visit was. The Medicare fees vary between $25 and $98, depending on the complexity of the visit, while private patients can pay up to $300 for a visit. Medicare and Medicaid have many other rules, as well, on such matters as maximum allowable charges, participating versus nonparticipating physicians, and so forth.

Many of the charges for Medicaid are so low that some physicians hesitate to care for these patients or decide to restrict the number of such patients they will see. Even Medicare fees are 30–50 percent lower than physicians' normal fees, and some physicians prefer not to accept new Medicare patients in their practice.

As health care expenditures have soared, state and federal governments have instituted such cost-containment tools as DRGs and utilization review:

DRGs. State and federal governments have sought to control costs by instituting a new schedule of payments to hospitals. These are known as diagnosis related groupings, or DRGs. In this system, every possible illness and procedure is assigned a dollar amount and a proposed length of stay (LOS). Your admission diagnosis determines how much the hospital is paid for your hospitalization and how many days you spend in the hospital.

In the past, hospitals were reimbursed for each day of a patient's stay, regardless of the diagnosis. Today, hospitals are paid the same amount whether you stay for two or twenty days. Clearly, the goal of DRGs is to encourage hospitals to shorten the length of your stay. Every hospital day that is eliminated saves the insurer—in this case, the government—a great deal of money.

For example, Ms. Jones has her gallbladder removed. The approved LOS for this DRG (cholecystectomy) is five days. If Ms. Jones is discharged on the third day after her surgery, the hospital is paid the same amount of money that it would have received if she had stayed the full five days. The hospital wins a minor victory (and even gets to be paid "twice" for the same hospital bed if another patient uses it for those two days). However, if Ms. Jones has a postoperative complication, is transferred into the intensive care unit, and is not discharged until seventeen days after her operation, the hospital is still reimbursed on the basis of a five-day DRG. So now the "victory" is the government's, not the hospital's.

How do DRGs affect patients? At times, the attending physician or the utilization reviewer (see below) may feel that the patient is ready for discharge—but if the patient elects to stay longer, he or she is responsible for the total cost of the additional days. With daily hospital charges in metropolitan areas averaging over $1,000, this can be quite costly. For example, Ms. Jones, who had her gallbladder removed, is eighty-six years old. After five days (the declared length of stay for this DRG), her daily occupancy of a hospital bed costs the hospital $500. When her physician declares her medically fit to go home, it turns out to be on a Friday. Her children, both of whom are working, ask the hospital to postpone the discharge until Saturday, when they can pick her up and help care for her at home. The hospital refuses and informs the distraught family that it will cost them $500 for the extra day.

Utilization Review. In order to speed patient flow, hospitals have created a "policing bureaucracy" known as utilization review, or regulatory affairs. Most utilization reviewers are nurses hired to read patients' charts on a daily basis. If they feel that the patient is ready for discharge, or that the pace of the testing or therapy is too slow, they act in the hospital's interest to speed things along. Reviewers can expedite tests so that they are done immediately, rather than on a first-come, first-served basis. They can pressure a surgeon to move up a case in his/her schedule, or pressure the administrators to make more operating time available for the case.

For example, let's say that Mr. Vasquez is admitted for a cardiac catheterization to ascertain the extent of his arteriosclerosis. The test makes it clear that he needs cardiac bypass surgery—and soon; it is not safe to send him home to be readmitted at a later date for the operation. The problem is that the cardiac surgeon has elective cases booked for the entire next week. Mr. Vasquez languishes in his hospital bed for two days waiting to see the surgeon. The reviewer, noting the delay, calls the hospital administrator, who calls the surgeon's office and insists on "bumping" an elective outpatient from the schedule to make room for Mr. Vasquez. Utilization review is also practiced by some private insurance plans.

■ ■ ■

Additional cost-containment measures will probably be developed as well. For example, currently, Medicare and Medicaid patients can be admitted to the hospital of their choice. But recent trends indicate that government-sponsored insurance plans may some day require admission to specific hospitals.

HMOs

HMOs are Health Maintenance Organizations, considered by some to be the wave of the future. HMO members pay a fixed amount of money per year for their medical insurance, which covers all costs of their care for that year, whether for an office visit for an upset stomach or hospitalization for cardiac surgery. HMO members who need to be hospitalized are only permitted to use those hospitals with which their HMO has a contract.

Members who are healthy and require few services generate income for the HMO, while those who require a great deal of care cost the HMO money.

Not all HMOs are financially or physically organized in the same manner. In some HMOs, doctors are HMO employees, all work in the same center, and are expected to see a minimum number of patients each week. Their compensation is fixed, however, so there is no incentive or disincentive to order tests. Any special or expensive tests they order may have to be approved by an administrator, who is obviously more concerned about the bottom line.

In other HMOs, family physicians are paid a yearly fee for each patient in their "panel" (group). They get the same fee whether they see a patient once or one hundred times. If all their patients stay healthy and rarely need to be seen, they receive their salary for little work. If their patients are very sick, they may do a lot of work for relatively low compensation.

Some of these plans have built-in disincentives for family physicians who order multiple tests or frequently hospitalize their patients: Any time a patient is referred to a specialist or has expensive tests performed, the cost may be deducted from the payment made to the family physician by the HMO. The HMO thus makes the family physician a "gatekeeper" who has a vested interest in *not* referring to specialists or ordering certain tests. Fortunately, such plans have become less common as both patients and physicians have found the concept distasteful.

Clearly, the gatekeeper system is biased toward rendering less care to more people. Although perhaps a cost-efficient system, the HMO unfortunately pits profit against traditional standards of patient care. Furthermore, by attempting to enroll only the healthiest patients, HMOs may place further strain on the other types of medical insurance plans by leaving them the sickest patients to care for.

MANAGED CARE

Managed care is the vogue concept of the 1990s as far as health insurance coverage is concerned. It applies the notion of supply-side economics to health insurance by positing that large groups of patients can use their combined financial clout to bargain with hospitals and physicians for lower prices.

In essence, the administrators of a managed-care plan (businesspeople who may or may not be physicians) negotiate the cheapest rates possible for medical care with hospitals and health care providers. All visits and procedures are covered—but you may "get what you pay for." In a worst-case scenario, managed care could turn medicine into an impersonal, cost-driven, assembly-line business, where doctors will see the most patients in the shortest amount of time, and hospitals will offer the most minimal care.

To a patient, what is most important is freedom of choice, quality, convenience, and availability. To a managed-care administrator, the bottom line is money, money, money. Managed-care contracts only work if they can get things done cheaply. Generalists replace specialists. Nurses replace physicians. Hospital admissions are replaced by ambulatory procedures, and as with HMOs, patients can only be admitted to specific participating hospitals.

WORKERS' COMPENSATION

Workers' (formerly workmen's) compensation, an insurance plan that employers are required by law to provide for employees, covers any job-related injury or illness. For example, it covers work-related trauma (a piece of machinery fell on your leg) or exposure to toxins (you work in a dry-cleaning store and have been overcome by fumes). Both full-time and part-time workers are covered for doctor's-office visits and hospitalization.

HOSPITAL CHARGES

When a hospital bill finally arrives, it seems to be in gibberish, listing pages and pages of charges for things that you have no hope of understanding. Despite the language barrier, it is a good idea to tackle the thing and try to interpret it. Because of the complexities of medical billing, most hospital accounts (some studies estimate 100 percent of them) contain errors, and in the end, we all pay for it.

Additionally, many charges appear that seem to have no basis in reality. Why does a day in a hospital bed cost $750? You had your gallbladder out, and required only minimal attention. Nurses came into your room just to give you occasional pain medications or check your temperature. For $750 a day, you could have had a suite at a deluxe hotel and round-the-clock butler service!

You are right to protest. It did not cost the hospital $750 a day to provide you with your care. However, Ms. McGillicuddy in the room down the hall cost the hospital $1,500 a day and her insurance paid the same $750. Your $750 helps the hospital to subsidize her care.

There are other factors that add to the daily cost per room. For example, every aspect of hospital care costs more money because of liability issues. Also, when a company produces medical equipment, it has a limited market, therefore the cost per unit is higher to cover research and development and to make a reasonable profit.

Another oddity you may notice on the bill is that all services and procedures are charged for separately. This contributes to the bill's length and complexity. There are separate charges for the operating room, for the recovery room, for every blood test, IV, and pill. There is no way after a long hospitalization that you can possibly remember every test you had and every medication you received. Why is it billed this way? The hospitals have learned that insurance companies will pay more for each separate test than for a clump of tests.

Why did you have so many blood tests anyway? The doctors did not have any financial incentive to order these tests. One reason is that medical students in this country are taught to cover all eventualities by doing as many tests as possible. This is reinforced by physicians' fear of malpractice suits. Although some studies by trial-lawyer associations report that malpractice fears do not contribute to the higher cost of medicine, most practicing physicians would admit that many tests are ordered just as protection against the possibility of future litigation.

Despite the complications of medical insurance and the complexities of hospital bills, the "bottom line" is that the United States has the best medical care system in the world when compared fairly with any other country. That's why many wealthy foreign nationals come here for their medical care. Whatever changes may be made in the country's health care policies and plans, it is hoped that all Americans—regardless of age, socioeconomic status, or medical condition—can have access to high-quality medical care.

SCHEDULE OF RATES
(Average room rates in New York City)

DAILY ROOM CHARGES	PRIVATE	SEMI-PRIVATE
MAIN HOSPITAL		
	$1,444.00 to $1,628.00	$968.00
Pediatrics	$1,444.00	$968.00
Pediatric Single Room		$1,265.00
Intensive Care Units	$2,051.00 to $2,516.00	
Special Care Units	$2,051.00, $2,283.00 to $2,516.00	
Coronary Care Unit		$1,819.00
Neonatal Intensive Care Center		$1,819.00
Neonatal Intermediate Care Center		$1,625.00
Neonatal Special Care Center		$1,345.00
Burn and Trauma Center		$2,237.00
LYING-IN HOSPITAL		
Gynecology	$1,231.00	$968.00
Obstetrics	$1,231.00	$968.00
Newborn Nursery		$500.00
OTHER CHARGES		
Isolation Surcharge	$150.00	
Operating Room		
(varies by procedure and time)	$1,082.00 to $15,509.00	
Postoperative Service (Recovery Room)	$300.50 to $4,629.00	
Delivery Room (normal delivery)	$527.00	

IMPORTANT INFORMATION ABOUT YOUR HOSPITAL FEES

Physician's Fee
The fees for your personal physician, surgeon, anesthesiologist, or consultant are not included in your hospital charges. They are considered a private agreement between you and your physician with billing and payment handled on a direct and personal basis. PLEASE DIRECT ANY QUESTIONS YOU MAY HAVE TO THE INDIVIDUAL PHYSICIAN CONCERNED.

Deposits
Patients who do not have insurance or those whose insurance plans do not accept full responsibility for hospital services provided will be asked to

pay a deposit toward their bill for each week of estimated stay at the time of admission. Obstetrical patients not covered by hospitalization must pay a deposit in advance of admission. If insurance coverage is available for the mother only, a deposit is required for the nursery charges. Patients requesting private rooms are responsible for the difference between the most common semi-private room rate and the rate of the private room. Your insurance company may require precertification before you are admitted to a hospital for a non-emergency admission. It is also possible that your insurer may require a second physician's opinion for a surgical admission and notification within forty-eight hours after an emergency admission. Your insurance company may also limit the number of days you may stay in the hospital depending upon your illness, require that you pay a deductible, and/or cover only a percentage of the cost for the first few days of your hospital stay. If you are not sure about these requirements, we suggest that you contact your employer or insurance carrier directly, and inform your physician. Our Admitting Office and Patients Accounts staff are available should you need further assistance.

Billing
Your hospital bill includes a basic daily charge which covers your room, meals, and routine nursing care. All services for ancillary care such as X rays, laboratory tests, drugs, operating room and delivery room fees, when required, are additional.

Diagnostic Related Groups (DRGS)
In this state, the amount the hospital bills and receives from your primary insurance carrier, including Medicare, is based on the diagnosis and procedures you received while hospitalized. This amount, based on the Diagnostic Related Group (DRG), is established by law. The bills you receive will be an itemized list of all services and supplies given you during your stay. However, the amount the hospital receives is based on the diagnosis and procedures you received while hospitalized. This amount is established by the state department of health, and is not related to specific charges on the bill.

Payment
A final hospital bill, reflecting payments and charges, is available approximately 10 days after discharge. By paying your portion of the hospital bill promptly, you hold down the cost of health care. The hospital depends upon your prompt payment to meet financial obligations.

Credit Cards
We will accept payment of your portion of any hospital bill in excess of $10.00 by MasterCard, Visa, and American Express.

MEDICAL BILL

CHARGE CODE	DATE	CHARGE DESCRIPTION	AMOUNT COVERAGE	ESTIMATED INS.* PATIENT	DUE FROM
12011200	04/24/94	DAILY RATE INTENSIVE F042204	1,950.00		.00
12020042	04/24/94	EMERG VISIT	276.25		.00
12120003	04/24/94	DIFFERENTIAL	13.25		.00
12120018	04/24/94	PLATELET COUNT	20.25		.00
12120034	04/24/04	PROTHROMBIN TIME	18.00		.00
12120051	04/24/94	P.T.T.	27.25		.00
12120087	04/24/94	CBC W/O DIFFERENTIAL	14.25		.00
12120102	04/24/94	URINALYSIS-MICRO	6.50		.00
12120109	04/24/94	URINALYSIS W/O MICRO	14.25		.00
12210005	04/24/94	AMYLASE	19.25		.00
12210010	04/24/94	CALCIUM-BLOOD	15.25		.00
12210013	04/24/94	ELECTROLYTE SERIES	27.25		.00
12210017	04/24/94	CREATININE-BLOOD	18.00		.00
12210031	04/24/94	PH BLD-CO2 PO2 PCO2	109.25		.00
12210032	04/24/94	GLUCOSE (FBS)	13.25		.00
12210036	04/24/94	UREA NITROGEN (BUN)	14.25		.00
12210127	04/24/94	CPK ISOENZYME	57.25		.00
12210130	04/24/94	BIOCHEM ADM PROFILE	30.25		.00
12210200	04/24/94	SPEC HANDL LAB	8.25		.00
12210200	04/24/94	SPEC HANDL LAB	8.25		.00
12210200	04/24/94	SPEC HANDL LAB	8.25		.00
12210200	04/24/94	SPEC HANDL LAB	8.25		.00
12210200	04/24/94	SPEC HANDL LAB	8.25		.00
12280619	04/24/94	TYPE AND SCREEN BATTERY	33.25		.00
12300186	04/24/94	EMER CARE NEW COMPRE	177.00		.00
12450901	04/24/94	PORTABLE CHEST 1 VIEW	167.00		.00
12500000	04/24/94	FORMULARY DRUGS	5.00		.00
12500000	04/24/94	FORMULARY DRUGS	34.50		.00
12011200	04/25/94	DAILY RATE INTENSIVE F042204	1,950.00		.00
12120003	04/25/94	DIFFERENTIAL	13.25		.00
12120018	04/25/94	PLATELET COUNT	20.25		.00
12120034	04/25/94	PROTHROMBIN TIME	18.00		.00
12120034	04/25/94	PROTHROMBIN TIME	18.00		.00
12120034	04/25/94	PROTHROMBIN TIME	18.00		.00
12120051	04/25/94	P.T.T.	27.25		.00
12120051	04/25/94	P.T.T.	27.25		.00
12120051	04/25/94	P.T.T.	27.25		.00
12120087	04/25/94	CBC W/O DIFFERENTIAL	14.25		.00
12210127	04/25/94	CPK ISOENZYME	57.25		.00
12210127	04/25/94	CPK ISOENZYME	57.25		.00
12210127	04/25/94	CPK ISOENZYME	57.25		.00
12210127	04/25/94	CPK ISOENZYME	57.25		.00
12210130	04/25/94	BIOCHEM ADM PROFILE	30.25		.00
12210145	04/25/94	MINI-DIAG PROFILE	27.25		.00
12210200	04/25/94	SPEC HANDL LAB	8.25		.00
12210200	04/25/94	SPEC HANDL LAB	8.25		.00
12210200	04/25/94	SPEC HANDL LAB	8.25		.00
12210200	04/25/94	SPEC HANDL LAB	8.25		.00
12280619	04/25/94	TYPE AND SCREEN BATTERY	33.25		.00
12430001	04/25/94	ECG (12 LEAD)	64.25		.00
12500000	04/25/94	FORMULARY DRUGS	57.47		.00
12011200	04/26/94	DAILY RATE INTENSIVE F042204	1,950.00		.00
12040010	04/26/94	PHLEBTOMY	6.50		.00
12120003	04/26/94	DIFFERENTIAL	13.25		.00
12120018	04/26/94	PLATELET COUNT	20.25		.00
12120051	04/26/94	P.T.T.	27.25		.00
12120087	04/26/94	CBC W/O DIFFERENTIAL	14.25		.00
12210127	04/26/94	CPK ISOENZYME	57.25		.00
12210129	04/26/94	LDH ISOENZYME	60.00		.00
12210145	04/26/94	MINI-DIAG PROFILE	27.25		.00
12280619	04/26/94	TYPE AND SCREEN BATTERY	33.25		.00
12430001	04/26/94	ECG (12 LEAD)	64.25		.00
12500000	04/26/94	FORMULARY DRUGS	3.64		.00
12500000	04/26/94	FORMULARY DRUGS	68.57		.00

CHARGE CODE	DATE	CHARGE DESCRIPTION	AMOUNT	ESTIMATED INS.*	DUE FROM
			COVERAGE	PATIENT	
12011200	04/27/94	DAILY RATE INTENSIVE F042204	1,950.00		.00
12040001	04/27/94	PHLEBTOMY	6.50		.00
12120003	04/27/94	DIFFERENTIAL	13.25		.00
12120003	04/27/94	DIFFERENTIAL	13.25		.00
12120018	04/27/94	PLATELET COUNT	20.25		.00
12120018	04/27/94	PLATELET COUNT	20.25		.00
12120034	04/27/94	PROTHROMBIN TIME	18.00		.00
12120034	04/27/94	PROTHROMBIN TIME	18.00		.00
12120051	04/27/94	P.T.T.	27.25		.00
12120051	04/27/94	P.T.T.	27.25		.00
12120087	04/27/94	CBC W/O DIFFERENTIAL	14.25		.00
12120087	04/27/94	CBC W/O DIFFERENTIAL	14.25		.00
12210013	04/27/94	ELECTROLYTE SERIES	27.25		.00
12210017	04/27/94	CREATININE-BLOOD	18.00		.00
12210025	04/27/94	MAGNESIUM	31.50		.00
12210032	04/27/94	GLUCOSE (FBS)	13.25		.00
12210036	04/27/94	UREA NITROGEN (BUN)	14.25		.00
12210200	04/27/94	SPEC HANDL LAB	8.25		.00
12210200	04/27/94	SPEC HANDL LAB	8.25		.00
12210200	04/27/94	SPEC HANDL LAB	8.25		.00
12410003	04/27/94	CINEANGIOCARDIOGRAMS	252.25		.00
12410004	04/27/94	CARDIAC CATH L/H	1,876.50		.00
12410005	04/27/94	CORONARY ARTERIOGRAM	455.75		.00
12410016	04/27/94	P.T.C.A.	3,752.50		.00
12410016	04/27/94	P.T.C.A	3,752.50		.00
12430001	04/27/94	ECG (12 LEAD)	64.25		.00
12430001	04/27/94	ECG (12 LEAD)	64.25		.00
12430001	04/27/94	ECG (12 LEAD)	64.25		.00
12500000	04/27/94	FORMULARY DRUGS	13.12		.00
12500000	04/27/94	FORMULARY DRUGS	16.92		.00
12011200	04/28/94	DAILY RATE INTENSIVE F042204	1,950.00		.00
12120003	04/28/94	DIFFERENTIAL	13.25		.00
12120018	04/28/94	PLATELET COUNT	20.25		.00
12120087	04/28/94	CBC W/O DIFFERENTIAL	14.25		.00
12210013	04/28/94	ELECTROLYTE SERIES	27.25		.00
12210017	04/28/94	CREATININE-BLOOD	18.00		.00
12210032	04/28/94	GLUCOSE (FBS)	13.25		.00
12210036	04/28/94	UREA NITROGEN (BUN)	14.25		.00
12210127	04/28/94	CPK ISOENZYME	57.25		.00
12210127	04/28/94	CPK ISOENZYME	57.25		.00
12280619	04/28/94	TYPE AND SCREEN BATTERY	33.25		.00
12430001	04/28/94	ECG (12 LEAD)	64.25		.00
12530016	04/28/94	CANNULAE NASAL	112.25		.00
12500000	04/28/94	FORMULARY DRUGS	15.28		.00
12500000	04/28/94	FORMULARY DRUGS	16.17		.00
12011200	04/29/94	DAILY RATE INTENSIVE F042204	1,950.00		.00
12040001	04/29/94	PHLEBTOMY	6.50		.00
12120003	04/29/94	DIFFERENTIAL	13.25		.00
12120034	04/29/94	PROTHROMBIN TIME	18.00		.00
12120034	04/29/94	PROTHROMBIN TIME	18.00		.00
12120051	04/29/94	P.T.T.	27.25		.00
12120051	04/29/94	P.T.T.	27.25		.00
12120087	04/29/94	CBC W/O DIFFERENTIAL	14.25		.00
12210013	04/29/94	ELECTROLYTE SERIES	27.25		.00
12210017	04/29/94	CREATININE-BLOOD	18.00		.00
12210032	04/29/94	GLUCOSE (FBS)	13.25		.00
12210036	04/29/94	UREA NITROGEN (BUN)	14.25		.00
12210127	04/29/94	CPK ISOENZYME	57.25		.00
12210129	04/29/94	LDH ISOENZYME	60.00		.00
12430001	04/29/94	ECG (12 LEAD)	64.25		.00
12530016	04/29/94	CANNULAE NASAL	112.25		.00
12500000	04/29/94	FORMULARY DRUGS	11.50		.00
12500000	04/29/94	FORMULARY DRUGS	15.28		.00
12010100	04/30/94	DAILY RATE SEMI-PRVT F020602	968.00		.00
12040001	04/30/94	PHLEBTOMY	6.50		.00
12120034	04/30/94	PROTHROMBIN TIME	18.00		.00
12120051	04/30/94	P.T.T.	27.25		.00
12430001	04/30/94	ECG (12 LEAD)	64.25		.00

CHARGE CODE	DATE	CHARGE DESCRIPTION	AMOUNT COVERAGE	ESTIMATED INS.* PATIENT	DUE FROM
12530016	04/30/94	CANNULAE NASAL	112.25		.00
12500000	04/30/94	FORMULARY DRUGS	11.50		.00
12500000	04/30/94	FORMULARY DRUGS	11.50		.00
12500000	04/30/94	FORMULARY DRUGS	16.02		.00
12010100	05/01/94	DAILY RATE SEMI-PRVT F020602	968.00		.00
12040001	05/01/94	PHLEBTOMY	6.50		.00
12120034	05/01/94	PROTHROMBIN TIME	18.00		.00
12120051	05/01/94	P.T.T.	27.25		.00
12120087	05/01/94	CBC W/O DIFFERENTIAL	14.25		.00
12180026	05/01/94	SONO EXTR W1 DOPLER-ARTERIA	126.25		.00
12430001	05/01/94	ECG (12 LEAD)	64.25		.00
12530016	05/01/94	CANNULAE NASAL	112.25		.00
12500000	05/01/94	FORMULARY DRUGS	1.48		.00
12500000	05/01/94	FORMULARY DRUGS	8.07		.00
12010100	05/02/94	DAILY RATE SEMI-PRVT F020602	968.00		.00
12040001	05/02/94	PHLEBTOMY	6.50		.00
12120003	05/02/94	DIFFERENTIAL	13.25		.00
12120018	05/02/94	PLATELET COUNT	20.25		.00
12120034	05/02/94	PROTHROMBIN TIME	18.00		.00
12120051	05/02/94	P.T.T.	27.25		.00
12120087	05/02/94	CBC W/O DIFFERENTIAL	14.25		.00
12210013	05/02/94	ELECTROLYTE SERIES	27.25		.00
12210017	05/02/94	CREATININE-BLOOD	18.00		.00
12210032	05/02/94	GLUCOSE (FBS)	13.25		.00
12210036	05/02/94	UREA NITROGEN (BUN)	14.25		.00
12430001	05/02/94	ECG (12 LEAD)	64.25		.00
12530016	05/02/94	CANNULAE NASAL	112.25		.00
12500000	05/02/94	FORMULARY DRUGS	2.87		.00
12530016	05/03/94	CANNULAE NASAL	112.25		.00
12530016	05/03/94	CANNULAE NASAL	112.25		.00
12530016	05/03/94	CANNULAE NASAL	112.25		.00
12500000	05/03/94	FORMULARY DRUGS	5.05		.00
12500000	05/03/94	FORMULARY DRUGS	5.05		.00
		SUBTOTAL OF CHARGES	29,781.49	29,781.49	.00
12700000	05/06/94	COMMERICAL INS AUTO ALLOW	5,580.37	5,580.37	
12700000	05/06/94	COMMERICAL INS AUTO ALLOW	5,580.37-	5,580.37-	
		TOTAL CHARGES & EST. INSURANCE	29,781.49	29,781.49	.00

*INSURANCE COVERAGES ARE ESTIMATED AND ARE SUBJECT TO CHANGE.
IF THERE ARE ANY QUESTIONS CONCERNING THIS BILL, PLEASE CALL YOUR
INSURANCE COMPANY.

PLEASE PAY THIS AMOUNT   0.00

SUMMARY OF MEDICAL BILL

CHARGE CODE	DATE	CHARGE DESCRIPTION	AMOUNT COVERAGE	ESTIMATED INS.* PATIENT	DUE FROM
		SUMMARY OF CHARGES			
		SUMMARY ROOM & BOARD			
001		DAILY RATE INTENSIVE CARE 6 DAYS AT 1,950.00	11,700.00	11,700.00	
001		DAILY RATE SEMIPRIVATE 3 DAYS AT 968.00	2,904.00	2,904.00	
		SUBTOTAL ROOM & BOARD	14,604.00	14,604.00	.00
		SUMMARY ANCILLARY SERVICES			
127		ULTRASOUND	126.25	126.25	
236		EMERGENCY	453.25	453.25	
415		DRUGS	318.99	318.99	
421		LABORATORY-CLINICAL	2,482.00	2,482.00	
429		ECG	642.50	642.50	
431		CARDIAC CATHERIZATION	10,089.50	10,089.50	
432		RADIOLOGY	167.00	167.00	
442		RESPIRATORY THERAPY	898.00	898.00	
		SUBTOTAL ANCILLARY	15,177.49	15,177.49	
		TOTAL CHARGES & EST. INSURANCE	29,781.49	29,781.49	.00

*INSURANCE COVERAGES ARE ESTIMATED AND ARE SUBJECT TO CHANGE.
IF THERE ARE ANY QUESTIONS CONCERNING THIS BILL, PLEASE CALL YOUR
INSURANCE COMPANY.   PLEASE PAY THIS AMOUNT   0.00

CHAPTER 6

PATIENTS' RIGHTS

Increasingly, patients are becoming more involved in their own care, asking questions, comparison shopping, and making their wishes on a wide variety of issues known in advance of their hospitalization. Some physicians see this as an erosion of their authority, and, in fact, it is. Physicians are no longer the omnipotent decision makers of yesteryear, using their judgment to determine who is treated and who is not. While it might be argued that with their experience and training, doctors are in a better position to make life and death decisions, life is not only about objectivity and percentages. It is also about people's personalities, religious beliefs, and individual approaches to illness and death. "Patients' rights" refers to protective mechanisms that give people control over their own life—and sometimes even their death.

INFORMED CONSENT

"Informed consent" is the principle of assuring that medical or surgical treatments are given only when a person understands and agrees to them. Prior to giving informed consent, a person must receive an explanation of exactly what is going to occur, why the procedure is being done, what other options are available, and what the potential risks are of doing the procedure, of delaying the procedure, or of not doing it at all. After this discussion, the patient or a legal guardian signs a form stating that all the necessary information has been presented and understood.

Informed consent is required for both major procedures such as surgery and relatively minor procedures such as a spinal tap. A patient may withdraw consent at any time, even just before a procedure is performed. If a patient is incapacitated, legally incompetent (for example, mentally retarded), or a minor, the immediate family may give consent. In the presence of a witness, it may even be possible to give consent by phone.

Some minors may, by law, give consent on their own. For example, depending on state law, "emancipated minors," minors who are pregnant or who are parents, and minors who have received special permission from a judge may not need to have a parent or guardian give consent.

"DO NOT RESUSCITATE" (DNR) ORDERS

Standard hospital policy is that the medical staff must assume that in case of a medical emergency every patient wants to have all life-sustaining measures performed unless the patient has given specific instructions to the contrary. The most commonly known instructions are DNR ("Do Not Resuscitate") orders. They specify that if the patient's breathing or heartbeat stops, no artificial means should be employed to maintain life.

A DNR order, for example, would rule out use of an endotracheal tube, a hollow tube inserted down the windpipe (trachea) in a patient who cannot breathe independently. The tube connects the patient to a respirator, an artificial breathing machine that delivers oxygen and other gases and breathes for the patient. Once hooked up, people may be kept alive indefinitely, even if they never regain the ability to breathe on their own. A brain-dead person can be kept breathing as long as the heart, liver, and other organs are still functioning. Add to the respirator a dialysis machine to function for the kidneys, a pacemaker to generate a heartbeat, intravenous fluids to provide nourishment, and a multitude of other tubes in and out of every part of the body, and a human being can be artificially kept alive by medical technology.

Such medical interventions are often temporary, and each alone, or in combination, can save lives. However, technology sometimes seems to be running amok, as patients with no hope of regaining meaningful life are kept alive. They may be kept alive because they belong to religions or sects that believe that everything must be done at all times to keep a patient alive, regardless of the circumstances, or because the patients (or family members when the patient is incapacitated) insist that everything be done, regardless of the medical reality.

When family members disagree about what should be done, time-consuming and expensive legal battles often ensue, causing untold heartache for all concerned—and prolonged suffering for the patient. It can be distressing to see a loved one die, so it is understandable that some family members cannot bear to let go, even when they know that the patient is hopelessly ill. Patients who make their wishes known in advance can spare their families the agony of deciding this matter for them.

LIVING WILL

What can you do to make sure that your desire to avoid excessive use of medical technology is heeded? First discuss your decision with your physician, then prepare a "living will." This document outlines exactly what and how much should be done in case of catastrophe. Living wills are generally drafted by attorneys, although there are "do-it-yourself" kits and books for those who want to write their own. Keep one copy with your regular will, and send another copy to your physician's office for your file.

Unfortunately, no document can cover every eventuality. Some living wills include unreasonable statements that reflect an individual's lack of understanding of the nuances and complexities of technological intervention. For example, a patient who regards a respirator as the ultimate in degradation and loss of control may state that he or she wishes *never* to be attached to one. However, there are many instances when respirators may be needed only for several hours or days, after which the patient then improves and can lead a fully normal life. Under these circumstances, with excellent hopes for a full recovery, a respirator should be employed—and a living will should be flexible enough to permit it.

It is also important to understand that a DNR order does not mean the end of the patient's care, but relates only to a specific emergency situation that may arise in the care of critically ill patients. Usually, a

DNR order is accompanied by detailed instructions about the patient's complete care, including the administration of antibiotics, pain medications, intravenous fluids, and other day-to-day requirements. Any or all of these treatments can be administered under a DNR order, or they can be withheld, depending on the patient's or family's wishes. For example, a DNR order may stipulate that neither electric shock to the heart nor a respirator should be used, but may still permit a patient to receive antibiotics and pain medications.

Pneumonia used to be known as the "old man's friend" because it was a frequent complication of illness in older, debilitated patients and a common and relatively gentle cause of death. Nowadays, with our vast armamentarium of antibiotics, families must make a decision as to whether to treat someone or not. For example, a patient who makes almost no progress two weeks after a major stroke has very little chance of a meaningful recovery. Should that person be kept alive, reduced to a life of total dependence, with no conscious thought? All patients and families must make their own decisions.

The "Do Not Resuscitate" discussion is frequently difficult to initiate. Some families order their doctors not to tell patients their diagnosis, much less discuss DNR. This is generally a terrible mistake. Most people know when their health is seriously jeopardized, and trying to hide this reality only keeps them from speaking about painful issues with those closest to them. The patient and family both try to spare the other's feelings, with the result that important words—such as *I love you, I'm sorry*, and *I'll miss you*—are never said.

Often, critically ill people who cannot truly comprehend the issues involved are deemed "incompetent" to make their own DNR decision. In these cases, two separate physicians must attest in writing to the patient's incompetence, and a family member, usually a spouse, may issue the DNR order. The signed DNR form is then placed on the front of the patient's hospital chart, and a DNR order for the nursing staff is written in the patient's order book. If a patient regains the ability to make his or her own decisions, the DNR order is rescinded in writing, and any new instructions to be followed are added.

Occasionally, DNR orders are mistakenly or willfully ignored by hospital personnel, resulting in the continued intubation of a patient on a respirator who had requested that it be disconnected. There are no specific guidelines or regulations to follow in these cases. Generally, if the family is in complete agreement, the respirator is quietly turned off and nature allowed to take its course.

HEALTH CARE PROXY

Many states have adopted a policy of advising patients at the time of their admission to the hospital, when they are presumably still in full control of their faculties, to sign a "health care proxy" that designates someone to make critical medical decisions in case the patient is incapacitated. This empowerment lasts only as long as patients cannot make their own decisions, and affects no other aspect of their lives (such as financial matters or child custody).

A health care proxy is very much like a limited power of attorney. Any individual—not only a relative—may be designated. On any subsequent hospital admissions, the proxy is considered null and void and must be specifically empowered again.

Choose your health care proxy carefully and discuss with your designee various strategies to cover as many eventualities as possible. Select a person whose judgment you trust completely and who you are sure will always act in your best interests. Make sure your proxy knows how you feel about advanced life support, DNR, organ donation and transplantation, and even abortion, in the event that you are pregnant.

There are other patients' rights to be aware of:

- You must understand the nature of your illness and the different treatment options.
- Nobody should coerce you into an experimental study.
- If you disagree with your treatment, you have the right to call in another physician to review it, and he or she must be granted full access to your medical record. The general protocol to follow: Tell your attending physician that you wish to get another opinion, and request that timely access be granted.
- If you do not agree with the date of discharge, you may dispute it.
- You may refuse any or all treatment. You may leave the hospital at any time, but you must sign a form stating that you are leaving against the advice of your physician.

In many states, a document listing patients' rights is prominently displayed within hospitals and given to each patient admitted electively. If you have any questions, ask to speak to the hospital's patient-services representative. These guardians of patients' rights are generally empathetic and have a great deal of experience in handling patients' problems and advocating on their behalf.

TWO PERSPECTIVES ON DNR ORDERS

"Do Not Resuscitate" orders reveal a great deal about individuals' perspectives and values.

Some people want to fight for life until the bitter end, regardless of the chance of success or the extreme measures that may be required. Perhaps they believe that life and death should be "in God's hands," and that God's will includes life support systems. Or they may harbor great reservoirs of hope and refuse to accept other people's hopelessness. Some people believe in miracles, or that life, whatever its trials, should be clung to and not let go.

In contrast are people who reject a fight that seems sure to be fruitless. Above all, they desire to avoid the great pain or loss of dignity that may accompany terminal conditions. Or they may feel, as do those mentioned above, that life and death should be in God's hands, but this group believes that God's will is that they should refuse life support systems. They may have exhausted their reservoirs of hope, and want to spare their families the torment of watching them suffer and the financial hardship of postponing inevitable death.

Both points of views are equally valid and to be respected. In such matters, there is no hard-and-fast "right or wrong," but rather the universal need to respect individuals' beliefs.

Appointing Your Health Care Agent

PROXY LAW

A new law called the health care proxy law allows you to appoint someone you trust—for example, a family member or close friend—to decide about treatment if you lose the ability to decide for yourself. You can do this by using a health care proxy form like the one inside, to appoint your "health care agent."

This law gives you the power to make sure that health care professionals follow your wishes. Your agent can also decide how your wishes apply as your medical condition changes. Hospitals, doctors, and other health care providers must follow your agent's decisions as if they were your own.

You can give the person you select, your health care agent, as little or as much authority as you want. You can allow your agent to decide about all health care or only certain treatments. You may also give your agent instructions that he or she has to follow.

Why should I choose a health care agent?

If you become too sick to make health care decisions, someone else must decide for you. Health care professionals often look to family members for guidance. But family members are not allowed to decide to stop treatment, even when they believe that is what you would choose or what is best for you under the circumstances. Appointing an agent lets you control your medical treatment by:

- allowing your agent to stop treatment when he or she decides that is what you would want or what is best for you under the circumstances;
- choosing one family member to decide about treatment because you think that person would make the best decisions or because you want to avoid conflict or confusion about who should decide; and
- choosing someone outside your family to decide about treatment because no one in your family is available or because you prefer that someone other than a family member decide about your health care.

How can I appoint a health care agent?

All competent adults can appoint a health care agent by signing a form called a Health Care Proxy. You don't need a lawyer, just two adult witnesses. You can use the form printed here, but you don't have to.

When would my health care agent begin to make treatment decisions for me?

Your health care agent would begin to make treatment decisions after doctors decide that you are not able to make health care decisions. As long as you are able to make treatment decisions for yourself, you will have the right to do so.

What decisions can my health care agent make?

Unless you limit your health care agent's authority, your agent will be able to make any treatment decision that you could have made if you were able to decide for yourself. Your agent can agree that you should receive treatment, choose among different treatments, and decide that treatments should not be provided, in accord with your wishes and interests. If your health care agent is not aware of your wishes about artificial nutrition and hydration (nourishment and water provided by feeding tubes), he or she will not be able to make decisions about these measures. Artificial nutrition and hydration are used in many circumstances, and are often used to continue the life of patients who are in a permanent coma.

How will my health care agent make decisions?

You can write instructions on the proxy form. Your agent must follow your oral and written instructions, as well as your moral and religious beliefs. If your agent does not know your wishes or beliefs, your agent is legally required to act in your best interests.

Who will pay attention to my agent?

All hospitals, doctors, and other health care facilities are legally required to honor the decisions by your agent. If a hospital objects to some treatment options (such as removing certain treatment) they must tell you or your agent in advance.

What if my health care agent is not available when decisions must be made?

You can appoint an alternate agent to decide for you if your health care agent is not available or able to act when decisions must be made. Otherwise, health care providers will make treatment decisions for you that follow instructions you gave while you were still able to do so. Any instructions that you write on your Health Care Proxy form will guide health care providers under these circumstances.

What if I change my mind?

It is easy to cancel the proxy, to change the person you have chosen as your health care agent, or to change any treatment instructions you have written on your Health Care Proxy form. Just fill out a new form. In addition, you can require that the Health Care Proxy expire on a specified date or if certain events occur. Otherwise, the Health Care Proxy will be valid indefinitely. If you choose your spouse as your health care agent and you get divorced or legally separated, the proxy is automatically canceled.

Can my health care agent be legally liable for decisions made on my behalf?

No. Your health care agent will not be liable for treatment decisions made in good faith on your behalf. Also, he or she cannot be held liable for costs of your care, just because he or she is your agent.

Is a health care proxy the same as a living will?

No. A living will is a document that provides specific instructions about health care treatment. It is generally used to declare wishes to refuse life-sustaining treatment under certain circumstances.

In contrast, the health care proxy allows you to choose someone you trust to make treatment decisions on your behalf. Unlike a living will, a health care proxy does not require that you know in advance all the decisions that may arise. Instead, your health care agent can interpret your wishes as medical circumstances change and can make decisions you could not have known would have to be made. The health care proxy is just as useful for decisions to receive treatment as it is for decisions to stop treatment. If you complete a Health Care Proxy form, but also have a living will, the living will provides instructions for your health care agent, and will guide his or her decisions.

Where should I keep the proxy form after it is signed?

Give a copy to your agent, your doctor, and any other family members or close friends you want. You can also keep a copy in your wallet or purse or with other important papers.

APPOINTING A HEALTH CARE AGENT IS A SERIOUS DECISION. MAKE SURE YOU TALK ABOUT IT WITH YOUR FAMILY, CLOSE FRIENDS, AND YOUR DOCTOR.

DO IT IN ADVANCE, NOT JUST WHEN YOU ARE PLANNING TO ENTER THE HOSPITAL.

About the Health Care Proxy

This is an important legal form. Before signing this form, you should understand the following facts:

1. This form gives the person you choose as your agent the authority to make all health care decisions for you, except to the extent you say otherwise in this form. "Health care" means any treatment, service, or procedure to diagnose or treat your physical or mental condition.

2. Unless you say otherwise, your agent will be allowed to make all health care decisions for you, including decisions to remove or withhold life-sustaining treatment.

3. Unless your agent knows your wishes about artificial nutrition and hydration (nourishment and water provided by a feeding tube), he or she will not be allowed to refuse those measures for you.

4. Your agent will start making decisions for you when doctors decide that you are not able to make health care decisions for yourself.

You may write on this form any information about treatment that you do not desire and/or those treatments that you want to make sure your receive. Your agent must follow your instructions (oral and written) when making decisions for you.

If you want to give your agent written instructions, do so right on the form. For example, you could say:

If I become terminally ill, I do/don't want to receive the following treatments: _____

If I am in a coma or unconscious, with no hope of recovery, then I do/don't want _____

If I have brain damage or a brain disease that make me unable to recognize people or speak and there is not hope that my condition will improve, I do/don't want _____

I have discussed with my agent my wishes about _____ *and I want my agent to make all decisions about these measures.*

Examples of medical treatments about which you may wish to give your agent special instructions are listed below. This is not a complete list of the treatments about which you may leave instructions.

- artificial respiration
- artificial nutrition and hydration (nourishment and water provided by feeding tube)
- cardiopulmonary resuscitation (CPR)
- antipsychotic medication
- electric shock therapy
- antibiotics
- psychosurgery
- dialysis
- transplantation
- blood transfusions
- abortion
- sterilization

Talk about choosing an agent with your family and/or close friends. You should discuss this form with a doctor or another health care professional, such as a nurse or social worker, before you sign it to make sure that you understand the types of decisions that may be made for you. You may also wish to give your doctor a signed copy. You do not need a lawyer to fill out this form.

You can choose any adult (over 18), including a family member, or close friend, to be your agent. If you select a doctor as your agent, he or she may have to choose between acting as your agent or as your attending doctor; a physician cannot do both at the same time. Also, if you are a patient or resident of a hospital, nursing home, or mental hygiene facility, there are special restrictions about naming someone who works for that facility as your agent. You should ask staff at the facility to explain those restrictions.

You should tell the person you choose that he or she will be your health care agent. You should discuss your health care wishes and this from with your agent. Be sure to give him or her a signed copy. Your agent cannot be sued for health care decisions made in good faith.

Even after you have signed this form, you have the right to make health care decisions for yourself as long as you are able to do so, and treatment cannot be given to you or stopped if you object. You can cancel the control given to your agent by telling him or her or your health care provider orally or in writing.

Filling Out the Proxy Form

Item (1) Write your name and the name, home address, and telephone number of the person you are selecting as your agent.

Item (2) If you have special instructions for your agent, you should write them here. Also, if you wish to limit your agent's authority in any way, you should say so here. If you do not state any limitations, your agent will be allowed to make all health care decisions that you could have made, including the decision to consent to or refuse life-sustaining treatment.

Item (3) You may write the name, home address, and telephone number of an alternate agent.

Item (4) This form will remain valid indefinitely unless you set an expiration date or condition for its expiration. This section is optional and should be filled in only if you want the health care proxy to expire.

Item (5) You must date and sign the proxy. If you are unable to sign yourself, you may direct someone else to sign in your presence. Be sure to include your address.

Two witnesses at least 18 years of age must sign your proxy. The person who is appointed agent or alternate agent cannot sign as a witness.

HEALTH CARE PROXY

(1) I, _____

hereby appoint _____
_(NAME, HOME ADDRESS, AND TELEPHONE NUMBER)

as my health care agent to make any and all health care decisions for me, except to the extent that I state otherwise. This proxy shall take effect when and if I become unable to make my own health care decisions.

(2) Optional instructions: I direct my agent to make health care decisions in accord with my wishes and limitations as stated below, or as he or she otherwise knows. (Attach additional pages if necessary.)

_____

_____

_____

(Unless your agent knows your wishes about artificial nutrition and hydration [feeding tubes], your agent will not be allowed to make decisions about artificial nutrition and hydration.

(3) Name of substitute or fill-in agent if the person I appoint above is unable, unwilling, or unavailable to act as my health care agent.

_____
_(NAME, HOME ADDRESS, AND TELEPHONE NUMBER)

(4) Unless I revoke it, this proxy shall remain in effect indefinitely, or until the date or conditions stated below. This proxy shall expire (specific date or conditions, if desired):

_____

(5) Signature _____

Address _____

Date _____

Statement by Witnesses (must be 18 or older)

I declare that the person who signed this document is personally known to me and appears to be of sound mind and acting of his or her own free will. He or she signed (or asked another to sign for him or her) this document in my presence.

Witness 1 _____

Address _____

Witness 2 _____

Address _____

Date _____

THE PATIENT'S BILL OF RIGHTS

The following Patient's Bill of Rights is strongly endorsed by the hospital on behalf of its patients. If you have any questions regarding any section or part of this statement of patient's rights, please contact the Administration Office, or write to the President of the hospital.

The patient is assured the right to:

1. Understand and use these rights. If for any reason you do not understand, or need help, the hospital must provide assistance, including an interpreter.

2. Receive emergency medical care, as indicated by the patient's medical condition, upon arrival at a hospital for the purpose of obtaining medical treatment.

3. Considerate and respectful care.

4. Upon request, obtain the name of the physician assigned the responsibility for coordinating his/her care; and the right to consult with his/her private physician and/or specialist for the type of care being rendered, provided such physician has been accorded hospital staff privileges.

5. The name and function of any person providing treatment to the patient.

6. Obtain from his/her physician complete current information concerning his/her diagnosis, treatment, and prognosis in terms the patient can be reasonably expected to understand. When it is not medically advisable to give such information to the patient, the information shall be made available to an appropriate person on the patient's behalf.

7. Receive from his/her physician information necessary to give informed consent prior to the start of any non-emergency procedure or treatment, or both (involving either non-emergency treatment, procedure, or surgery, or a diagnostic procedure which involves invasion or disruption of the integrity of the body). An informed consent shall include, as a minimum, the specific procedure or treatment or both, the reasonably foreseeable risks involved, and alternatives for care or treatment, if any, as a reasonable medical practitioner under similar circumstances would disclose.

8. Be informed that the right to consent to treatment includes the right to refuse treatment, including life-sustaining treatment to the extent permitted by law and to be informed of the medical consequences of your refusal to consent.

9. Be informed of your right to express your wishes and/or instructions with respect to treatment in advance of becoming unable to do so. This right may be exercised by designating an individual to make treatment decisions for you, creating a living will, consenting to a do not resuscitate order and/or taking other steps which clearly evidence your wishes regarding treatment.

10. Receive all the information you need to give informed consent for an order not to resuscitate. You also have the right to designate an individual to give this consent for you if you are too ill to do so.

11. Privacy while in the hospital and confidentiality of all information and records regarding your care.

12. Refuse to participate in research. Human experimentation affecting care or treatment shall be performed only with the patient's informed effective consent.

13. Examine and receive an explanation of his/her bill, regardless of source of payment.

14. Express complaints about the care and services provided, and to have the hospital investigate such complaints. The hospital is responsible for providing the patient or his/her designee with a written response if requested by the patient indicating the findings of the investigation. The hospital is also responsible for notifying the patient or his/her designee that if the patient is not satisfied by the hospital response, the patient may complain to the state department of health.

15. A smoke-free environment in all patient rooms and treatment areas. Patients who need to smoke based upon medical necessity may do so in designated areas provided for this purpose upon orders by the physician.

16. Treatment without discrimination as to age, race, color, religion, sex, sexual orientation, citizenship, national origin or source of payment, except for fiscal capability thereof. You also have the right not be discriminated against based upon whether or not you have expressed your wishes concerning your treatment in advance of your becoming unable to do so.

17. Review your medical record without charge and obtain a copy of your medical record for which the hospital can charge a reasonable fee. You cannot be denied a copy solely because you cannot afford to pay.

18. a) Prior to discharge from an inpatient service, receive an appropriate written patient discharge plan and a written description of the patient discharge review process available to the patient under federal or state law.

    b) A copy of the provisions of this section shall be given to each patient or the patient's appointed personal representative upon admission for treatment as an inpatient, outpatient and/or emergency room patient at, or up to 14 days prior to, the time of admission to the hospital and shall be posted in conspicuous places within the hospital.

DNR DOCUMENTATION: ADULT PATIENT WITH CAPACITY

Directions: This documentation sheet sets forth in consecutive order the steps that must be followed before writing a DNR ORDER for an ADULT patient with CAPACITY. Words that appear in all capital letter are defined in the DNR Policy. When completed, this sheet must be placed in the patient's medical record.

Step One

The ATTENDING PHYSICIAN must provide the patient with information regarding CPR and a DNR ORDER.

ATTENDING PHYSICIAN'S STATEMENT

Before the patient gave consent to a DNR ORDER, I provided to the patient information about his/her diagnosis and prognosis, the range of available resuscitation measures, the reasonably foreseeable risks and benefits of cardiopulmonary resuscitation for him/her, and the consequences of a DNR order.

_____
Signature of Attending Physician

_____
Print Name   M.D. Code

Date _____

Step Two

The patient must give oral or written consent to a DNR ORDER at or about the time the DNR ORDER is to be issued. Oral consent must be given during hospitalization in the presence of two WITNESSES, one of whom must be a physician on staff at the hospital.

WITNESSES' STATEMENT

The patient has expressed orally in my presence the decision to consent to a DNR ORDER, subject to the following conditions or limitations (if any):

_____
Signature of Witness

_____
Print Name

_____
Title/Relationship to Patient

Date _____

_____
Signature of Physician Witness

_____
Print Name   M.D. Code

Date _____

Instead of oral consent, the patient may choose to consent in writing to the DNR ORDER. Written consent must be dated and signed by the patient and two WITNESSES. A copy of the written consent must be placed in the medical record.

IF THE PATIENT IS IN OR IS TRANSFERRED FROM A MENTAL HYGIENE FACILITY SEE BELOW*

Step Three

The ATTENDING PHYSICIAN must promptly do one of the following:

a. issue the DNR ORDER, or issue the order at such time as any conditions specified in the patient's decision are met, and either write the order himself or herself or direct the house staff to do so; or

b. make his/her objections to the DNR ORDER and the reasons for those objections known to the patient and either transfer the patient to another ATTENDING PHYSICIAN or submit the matter to the DISPUTE MEDIATION SYSTEM.

Indicate action taken: (check one)

_____ DNR ORDER issued

_____ Patient transferred to another ATTENDING PHYSICIAN

_____ Matter submitted to DISPUTE MEDIATION SYSTEM

REMINDER: For inpatients, other than alternate level of care ("ALC") patients, the DNR ORDER must be reviewed every seven days, or sooner if there is an improvement in the patient's condition, and the review must be documented in the medical record. For ALC patients and outpatients, such review must be done each time the ATTENDING PHYSICIAN examines the patient, except that such review need not occur more than once every seven days. In addition, for ALC patients, the review must occur at least once every sixty days.

_____

* If the patient is in or is transferred from a MENTAL HYGIENE FACILITY, notice of the patient's consent to a DNR ORDER shall be given to the facility director prior to issuance of a DNR ORDER. Notification to the facility director shall not delay issuance of a DNR ORDER. If the facility director concludes that the patient lacks capacity or that issuance of a DNR ORDER may be inconsistent with the patient's wishes, the facility director shall submit the matter to the DISPUTE MEDIATION SYSTEM.

DNR DOCUMENTATION: ADULT PATIENT WITHOUT CAPACITY

Directions: This documentation sheet sets forth in consecutive order the steps that must be taken prior to writing a DNR ORDER for an ADULT patient without CAPACITY who has a HEALTH CARE AGENT. Words that appear in all capital letter are defined in the DNR Policy. When completed, this sheet must be placed in the patient's medical record.

Step One

The ATTENDING PHYSICIAN must determine that the patient lacks CAPACITY.

DETERMINATION OF CAPACITY

I have examined the patient and have determined to a reasonable degree of medical certainty that he/she lacks the ability to understand and appreciate the nature and consequences of a DNR ORDER, including the benefits and disadvantages, and to reach an informed decision. In my opinion, the cause and nature of the patient's incapacity is:

_____

and its extent and probable duration are: _____

_____

_____

_____
Signature of Attending Physician

_____
Print Name   M.D. Code

Date _____

Step Two

A CONCURRING PHYSICIAN must agree with the determination that the patient lacks capacity. (If the patient's incapacity is due to MENTAL ILLNESS, the concurring opinion must be provided by a physician who is certified by the American Board of Psychiatry and Neurology. If the patient's incapacity is due to a DEVELOPMENTAL DISABILITY, the concurring opinion must be provided by a physician with special credentials who has been designated by the Director of the Department of Psychiatry.)

CONCURRING PHYSICIAN'S STATEMENT

I have personally examined the patient and have determined to a reasonable degree of medical certainty that he/she lacks the ability to understand and appreciate the nature and consequences of a DNR ORDER, including the benefits and disadvantages, and to reach an informed decision. In my opinion, the cause and nature of the incapacity are:

_____

_____

_____

and its extent and probable duration are: _____

_____

_____
Signature of Concurring Physician

_____
Print Name   M.D. Code

Date _____

Step Three

The ATTENDING PHYSICIAN must notify the HEALTH CARE AGENT of the determination that the patient lacks CAPACITY. In addition, if there is any indication of the patient's ability to understand, notice must be given to the patient orally and in writing, together with a copy of the Department of Health's pamphlet, "Do Not Resuscitate Orders — A Guide for Patients and Families." If the patient is in or is transferred from a MENTAL HYGIENE FACILITY, notice must also be given to the facility director. Finally, notice must be given to a conservator or committee of the patient, if one has been appointed.

NOTICE TO PATIENT AND AGENT OF LACK OF CAPACITY

a)   I have given notice of the determination of the patient's lack of capacity to the agent:, and

b)   (Check one)

        _____   There is no indication of the patient's ability to comprehend such notice and I am therefore not giving notice to the patient; or

        _____   I have given the patient notice of the determination.

c)   (Check if applicable)

        _____   I have given notice to the mental hygiene facility director.

        _____   I have given notice to the patient's conservator/committee.

_____
Signature of Attending Physician

_____
Print Name   M.D. Code

Date _____

Step Four

The ATTENDING PHYSICIAN must provide the HEALTH CARE AGENT with information regarding CPR and a DNR ORDER.

ATTENDING PHYSICIAN'S STATEMENT

Before the patient's health care agent gave consent to a DNR ORDER, I provided to the agent information about the patient's diagnosis and prognosis, the range of available resuscitation measures, the reasonably foreseeable risks and benefits of cardiopulmonary resuscitation for the patient, and the consequences of a DNR ORDER.

_____
Signature of Attending Physician

_____
Print Name   M.D. Code

Date _____

Step Five

The HEALTH CARE AGENT must give oral or written consent to a DNR ORDER at or about the time the DNR ORDER is to be issued. Oral consent must be expressed to two WITNESSES, one of whom must be a physician on staff at the hospital.

WITNESSES' STATEMENT

The agent has expressed orally in my presence the decision to consent to a DNR ORDER, subject to the following conditions or limitations (if any):

_____

_____

_____
Signature of Witness

_____
Print Name

_____
Title/Relationship to Patient

Date _____

_____
Signature of Physician Witness

_____
Print Name   M.D. Code

Date _____

78

Instead of oral consent, the AGENT may choose to consent in writing to the DNR ORDER. Written consent must be dated and signed by the AGENT and two WITNESSES. A copy of the written consent must be placed in the medical record.

IF THE PATIENT OBJECTS, A DNR ORDER MUST NOT BE WRITTEN.

Step Six

The ATTENDING PHYSICIAN must promptly do one of the following:

a. issue the DNR ORDER, or issue the order at such time as any conditions specified in the AGENT'S decision are met, and either write the order himself or herself or direct the house staff to do so; or

b. make his/her objections to the DNR ORDER and the reasons for those objections known to the AGENT and either transfer the patient to another ATTENDING PHYSICIAN or submit the matter to the DISPUTE MEDIATION SYSTEM.

Indicate action taken: (check one)

_____ DNR ORDER issued

_____ Patient transferred to another ATTENDING PHYSICIAN

_____ Matter submitted to DISPUTE MEDIATION SYSTEM.

REMINDER: For inpatients, other than alternate level of care ("ALC") patients, the DNR ORDER must be reviewed every seven days, or sooner if there is an improvement in the patient's condition, and the review must be documented in the medical record. For all patients and outpatients, such review must be done each time the ATTENDING PHYSICIAN examines the patient, except that such review need not occur more than once every seven days. In addition, for ALC patients, the review must occur at least once every sixty days.

CHAPTER 7

THE ADMITTING OFFICE

U nless you arrive by am-
bulance, your first stop
upon entering the hos-
pital is the admitting office.
This is the business side of the
hospital, where you deal with
several types of paperwork.

IN A NUTSHELL

Preadmitting
Precertification
CPT and ICD-9 codes
Preadmission testing
Identification

PREADMITTING

For elective admissions, your physician's or surgeon's office will send the hospital a preadmission form.

The preadmission form contains medical information, including your diagnosis and any planned procedures, your vital statistics, and financial information. Before your admission is scheduled, the hospital and your insurance company must be in agreement about your diagnosis, treatment, and acceptable length of stay.

PRECERTIFICATION

Most insurance companies require you to call them for approval of an elective procedure before your admission to the hospital. You generally need to obtain the approval, called *precertification*, at least forty-eight hours prior to admission. When you call, be prepared to tell the insurance company: your insurance plan name and identification number(s); your *primary admission diagnosis*; the treatment or procedure your doctor has recommended.

If the insurance company approves your admission, it will give you a certification, precertification, or approval number, depending on the term your insurance company uses. Write down the number and give it to your doctor's secretary over the phone or in person.

If the insurance company does *not* give approval, this does not necessarily mean that your doctor has recommended inappropriate treatment. Perhaps the insurance company needs more information, or the doctor's recommendation differs with the company's policies (which are often guided more by the desire to cut costs than by concern for patients' comfort). For example, your doctor may want you to spend one night in the hospital after your cardiac catheterization. Your insurance company denies the overnight stay because according to their policy, the procedure is classified as an ambulatory (outpatient) procedure only.

When an insurance company denies approval, don't give up. You do have recourse.

Enlist your physician's help. Have your doctor's office call the insurance company to explain the need for the treatment, procedure, or overnight stay.

Conquer the insurance company's bureaucracy. If your doctor's call to the insurance company does not result in an approval, call the insurance company back and insist on speaking with a supervisor. If the supervisor continues to deny approval, demand to speak with the insurance company's doctor. *Be relentless!* Don't give up just because some lower-level bureaucrat says no. Work your way up through the layers of bureaucracy as far as you can go.

Coping with a stubborn insurance company can be difficult and time-consuming, giving you the feeling that the entire bureaucracy sprouted just to deny you your night in the hospital! If the insurance company continues to deny approval despite your best efforts, you can still proceed with the hospitalization, but will have to pay for it yourself.

An insurance company sometimes denies permission for an *inpatient* procedure, but allows you to receive treatment as an outpatient. However, if an emergency arises during your procedure and you must be admitted, your insurance company will pay for the inpatient admission.

The above concepts apply to *elective* (not emergency) admissions, which are generally surgical but may include certain elective medical admissions, such as a cardiac catheterization.

HOSPITAL NOTIFICATION

Many insurance companies require you to notify them of any admission—even an emergency or maternity admission—within a specified number of hours, usually twenty-four or forty-eight. Be familiar with the requirements of your insurance policy, which is often stated on the back of your insurance card.

Most medical admissions are not elective, but result from a referral from the emergency room. In an emergency, patients are admitted and cared for without any attempt to assess insurance coverage. Patients in the United States cannot be denied access to hospital care in an emergency, regardless of their ability to pay for their hospitalization.

CPT AND ICD-9 Codes

Hospitals, insurance companies, and physicians generally communicate with one another in code. These codes are arbitrary numbers known as the CPT (Common Procedural Terminology code) and the ICD-9 code (International Classification of Disease, revision 9). The CPT code refers to the procedure to be performed (e.g., removal of the gallbladder) and the ICD-9 code refers to your diagnosis (e.g., cholecystitis—inflamed gallbladder). For example, the CPT code 33510 and the ICD-9 code 414 indicate that a person is entering the hospital to have a cardiac bypass (CPT) because he had coronary artery disease

---

Claim Instructions

Hospitalization

In the event hospitalization becomes necessary —

- Present this card to the hospital admission clerk
- The hospital will submit data directly to health benefits.

All Other Care

A claim form must be submitted for all medical providers. Itemized bills for all covered expenses not included on the claim form should be attached to the claim form. These bills should show:

1. Name of patient
2. Nature of illness or injury
3. Type of Service

4. Date(s) service(s) rendered
5. Charge(s) made
6. Employee signature

For claims payments, coverage and eligibility information, call health benefits.

THIS IS NOT A HOSPITAL GUARANTEE CARD

(ICD-9). The CPT and ICD-9 codes must "go together." For example, if a diagnosis code indicates a hernia, and the procedure code indicates a breast biopsy, the insurance company denies approval of the hospitalization until it receives the correct concordance between codes.

The proper coding of the diagnosis and procedure is extremely important to you, not because it has any impact on your care, but because it can affect your insurance company's reimbursement to you, your physician, and the hospital. The coding also has a significant impact on the "length of stay," the amount of time that your insurance company allows you to stay in the hospital for each diagnosis and procedure. For example, if you are coded as having a urinary tract infection, the permitted length of stay is much shorter than the code for urinary sepsis. Many hospitals employ people whose sole function is to select the appropriate codes to maximize hospital reimbursement for a given illness, hospitalization, or set of diagnoses.

PREADMISSION TESTING

By now, the hospital and the insurance company have agreed upon your admission (you have been preapproved, or precertified). But don't pack your bags yet. Before most surgical and many medical admissions, appropriate testing must be done before the day you are actually admitted to the hospital. Testing may include an electrocardiogram (EKG), chest X ray, blood tests, and urine analysis. Tests can be done at your physician's office, or at a special outpatient section of the hospital. Only five or ten years ago, a patient was admitted to the hospital and had blood tests and X rays as an inpatient. But times have changed. Although inpatient testing is probably much more convenient for patients, it costs the government and your insurance company more money to admit patients the night before the procedure. Having the tests done before admission shortens the length of stay and permits cancellation of the procedure if anything irregular turns up, thus saving the insurance company the cost of the hospital day(s). (See Chapter 4, "Planning and Preparing for Surgery.")

Why would anyone wish to spend an extra night in the hospital? Imagine if you lived ninety minutes away and were required to be at the hospital by six in the morning. Imagine needing multiple enemas until your colon was all cleaned out. You would definitely appreciate that extra hospital night and the help from the nursing staff.

Prior to the present system, all the admission paperwork, initial history, and physical examination were done upon admission by an intern, resident, physician's assistant, or nurse practitioner. Now it is the responsibility of your physician's office to take care of this beforehand.

THE DAY BEFORE ADMISSION

The day before your scheduled admission, you will be contacted by a person in the admitting office to tell you what time to arrive in the hospital. However, just as airlines sometimes "overbook" a flight, you may find yourself "bumped." The number of available beds in a hospital changes hourly and is based upon planned discharges and the potential number of emergency admissions. Not all patients scheduled for discharge leave as planned. A complication may occur. A family member cannot pick up the patient until late in the afternoon. A bed planned for an elective admission may be needed for an emergency admission. All this can wreak havoc on admission-office personnel as they struggle to get people into the hospital—and may wreak havoc on your schedule, as well.

Most patients are discharged at ten or eleven in the morning, but just as in any hotel, the housekeeping department must then get the room clean and ready. So although the hospital tells you to come in at about one o'clock in the afternoon, there is always the chance that a bed may not be available because the patient in it is not going home as scheduled. In that case, you will be "bumped." Because hospitals have to run near 100 percent occupancy to stay solvent, they can no longer afford to keep a few beds open in reserve. This can mean a major inconvenience for you, but medicine is now unfortunately not only in the business of healing the sick but also in the business of staying in business.

THE BIG DAY

Like airports, admitting offices have large waiting rooms because now that you have arrived on schedule, you get to hurry up and wait. At last, you meet with the admission representative or officer. You are called into a small cubicle where you will go over all the information previously submitted. You must also decide on the type of room you will occupy (private or semiprivate), and consider whether you are willing to pay more out of your own pocket for a private room, since your insurer is highly unlikely to cover it. You may be asked to leave a deposit if you choose a private room. If the hospital *only* has a private room available, you may get it at semiprivate rates, but expect to be relocated when a semiprivate room becomes available.

Hospitals understand that the admitting office is an anxious place for a person about to become a patient, and try to staff it with "patient-friendly" workers.

IDENTIFICATION

A hospital's biggest nightmare is the possibility that the wrong procedure can be performed on the wrong patient. Over the years, a variety of safeguards have been instituted to correctly identify patients, including those who cannot identify themselves (e.g., because they are in a coma, are anesthetized, or are confused). The most important safeguard is the hospital identification number. Every admitted patient is assigned a number which remains with him or her as long as hospital records are kept (forever). This number is placed on every piece of paper associated with the patient, as well as directly on the person in the form of a wrist bracelet. This plastic identification tag is put on either in the admitting office, or as soon as the patient arrives on the floor. It is made to be very difficult to remove and contains, in most cases, the person's name and history number.

Additionally, many hospitals issue each patient a plastic card, much like a credit card, that can be used for identification. This card, unlike the wristband which is temporary and removed at the time of hospital discharge, may be carried and used indefinitely.

ADMIT: DAY SURGERY

PRE-ADMISSION TESTING AND HISTORY AND PHYSICAL FORM

(USE THIS FORM IF YOUR PATIENT WILL STAY OVERNIGHT ON THE DAY OF SURGERY)

PATIENT'S NAME	AGE
HISTORY NUMBER (UNCONFIRMED)	
PHYSICIAN'S NAME	NYH ID CODE
SURGICAL SERVICE	

(1) ADMISSION DIAGNOSIS	
(2) SECONDARY DIAGNOSIS	
(3) PROCEDURE/OPERATION	
PROCEDURE DATE	CONFIRMATION #
PRE-ADMISSION TEST DATE	☐ YES ☐ NO

TYPE OF ANESTHESIA PROPOSED:
☐ LOCAL
☐ MONITORED ANESTHESIA CARE
☐ GENERAL
☐ REGIONAL
☐ POST-OP PAIN CONSULT

FAMILY SUPPORT
☐ GOOD
☐ FAIR
☐ UNDETERMINED

SOCIAL WORK EVALUATION AVAILABLE

ALL TEST RESULTS MUST BE SUBMITTED 48 HOURS PRIOR TO SURGERY

PHYSICIAN'S ORDER SHEET

LABORATORY TESTS
☐ CBC
☐ CBC W/DIFF & PLATELETS
☐ PT/PTT
☐ BETAHCG - QUANT.
☐ UA W/MICRO
☐ OTHER:

☐ LYTES
☐ PREADMIT PROFILE
  (Lytes, BUN, Creat, Gluc)
☐ BIOCHEM PROFILE
☐ TYPE & SCREEN
☐ AUTOLOGOUS/DIRECTED
  BLOOD HAS BEEN
  APPROVED
☐ TYPE & CROSSMATCH
  (if blood is required for surgery)

DIAGNOSTIC TESTS:
☐ EKG
☐ CHEST X RAY

PRE-OPERATIVE ANTIBIOTIC PROPHYLAXIS ORDERS

ALLERGIES _____

TIME OF ADMINISTRATION _____

☐ AMPICILLIN 1 gram ivpb
☐ AMPICILLIN/SULBACTAM
  (Unasyn) 1.5 gram ivpb
☐ CEFAZOLIN 1 gram ivpb
☐ CEFOXITIN 1 gram ivpb
☐ DOXYCYCLINE
  100 mg ivpb

☐ GENTAMICIN (1.5 mg/kg ___
  mg ivpb)
☐ METRONIDAZOLE
  500 mg ivpb
☐ VANCOMYCIN 1 gram ivpb
  (should only be considered when patient has a penicillin allergy)

NOTE: Use of an antibiotic not listed above will require approval prior to use.

PHYSICIAN'S SIGNATURE

MD _____

DATE _____ MD CODE ☐☐☐☐☐

ANESTHESIOLOGY SECTION

ANESTHESIA CLEARANCE ☐ YES ☐ NO ☐ PENDING

PHYSICIAN NOTIFIED _____ TIME/DATE _____

TIME _____

PHYSICAL STATUS _____ RISK STATUS _____

CARDIOPULMONARY STATUS _____

_____
_____
_____
_____
_____
_____
_____
_____

ALLERGIES, MEDICATIONS & OTHER CONDITIONS _____

_____
_____
_____
_____
_____

ANESTHESIOLOGIST _____ DATE ____ CODE ____
(Signature)

CHAPTER 8

THE EMERGENCY ROOM

Television and movies tend to glorify the hospital emergency room (ER) as being an exciting, action-filled place—and often it is. When the ambulance pulls up and unloads drivers bloodied in a head-on collision, or a teenager with a gunshot wound, or a woman about to give birth, or a child with an unexplained seizure, the doctors, nurses, and other members of the ER team race to save their lives. Many things happen at once. While one physician inserts a breathing tube down the patient's throat, another starts an intravenous line, a nurse cuts away clothing that is in the way, and an orderly stands ready to help steer the gurney through the hall toward the operating room. Emergency room workers are often overworked; on a busy night, they may feel that their adrenaline never stops pumping.

But ER staff are also frustrated. Although they have expertise in responding to urgent medical matters, increasingly, people are misusing emergency rooms as ad hoc clinics for round-the-clock routine medical care. On the same night that ambulances seem to arrive every five minutes, the ER waiting room may be filled by a dozen people whose ailments are in quite a different league. An eight-year-old child has a fever and a cough. A middle-aged man who ate ancient potato salad from the back of his refrigerator has diarrhea, probably associated with mild food poisoning. A twenty-five-year-old man has been having burning sensations when he urinates; he and his girlfriend have come to the ER to find out if this might be a symptom of gonorrhea. All of them need medical attention, but could have waited until the next day to consult their private physician or clinic. By coming to the ER, they contribute to the long waits and congested conditions that complicate ER functioning and divert staff members' attentions from bona fide emergencies.

Emergency rooms are not allowed to refuse a patient treatment, so all comers must be seen. Individuals need to "prescreen" themselves, asking whether, indeed, an ailment is potentially serious enough to warrant a trip to the ER.

How do you know when you *should* go to the emergency room? Any illness that cannot be safely handled at home or in a physician's office requires an emergency room visit. This includes cardiac emergencies (heart attack), extensive trauma (such as a broken back, fractured skull, or ruptured spleen), strokes, severe infections, or sudden intractable pain. These situations are generally cared for in emergency rooms even during daylight hours when physicians are in their offices. It is safer to be treated in the ER where advanced life support equipment and trained emergency personnel are available at all times.

> **REASONS TO GO TO AN EMERGENCY ROOM**
>
> **On advice of a physician**
> **Severe chest pain**
> **Severe shortness of breath**
> **Bleeding**
> **Fainting**
> **Loss of consciousness**
> **Trauma**
> **High fever (over 101°)**
> **Stroke**
> **Dehydration**
> **Allergic reaction**
> **Poisoning**
> **Choking**

When told that they should go to the ER, some people are annoyed that physicians no longer seem to make house calls and insist on seeing them in the hospital. But it's important to remember that there are very few tests that can be done at home—whereas virtually all tests are instantly available in the ER. Electrocardiograms, chest X rays, complete blood counts, and other blood tests, as well as more complicated examinations (for example, a spinal tap) are available in the emergency room twenty-four hours a day.

Which emergency room should I go to?

This question has relevance for those who are lucky enough to live close to different types of hospitals. Hospitals that are designated as trauma centers have trained personnel to handle any type of serious accident and may be filled with accident victims at any time. If you are in a serious car accident and suffer multiple broken bones, this is a great place to be, because the care will be state of the art.

If you have a slightly less critical situation, such as a cut on the knee that requires stitches, you may be better off at a less busy ER where the care will be timely and less rushed, while still totally adequate for your needs.

Should I go to the ER by car or ambulance?

It depends on how ill you are. If you have time to speak to your doctor before leaving for the emergency room, ask for guidance as to whether to drive there or await the arrival of an ambulance.

Frequently, an ambulance is necessary for safe transportation to the ER. Standard ambulances are staffed by trained drivers and perhaps emergency medical technicians (EMT), and are primarily used for transportation and minor emergencies. Paramedic ambulances have personnel trained in advanced cardiac life support (ACLS) and trauma, and can provide treatment for a variety of life-threatening situations. Generally, the paramedics are in contact with emergency room physicians by shortwave radio so they can transmit patient data, including physical findings and electrocardiograms, for review and interpretation.

However you get to the ER, it is always best to have someone accompany you. Your companion can drive you if you don't need an ambulance, and can help you home if you are not quite sick enough to be admitted but are too sick to walk or drive yourself. He or she can take home your clothes and valuables if you are admitted, and provide crucial historical or medical information if you become incapacitated.

What happens when I arrive?

If you are critically ill and arrive by ambulance, you are almost always ushered right to the appropriate emergency room area for treatment. Emergency rooms within large hospitals generally have separate areas for the major specialties (surgery, internal medicine, pediatrics, obstetrics/gynecology, and psychiatry). In emergency situations, care is rendered first; forms can be filled out later.

If you are not acutely ill, your first stop will be at the registration desk. Here, you will be asked for such information as your address and phone number, date of birth, health insurance information, place of employment, physician's name, and any medications you are taking. (For more on such "vital statistics," see Chapter 3, "Consultation with a Surgeon.")

The next person you will see is the triage nurse. Triage is a system of priorities designed to maximize the number of survivors. The triage nurse is responsible for assessing the severity of your illness based on your description of symptoms or the appearance of your injury, and ensuring that the sickest patients are treated first. For example, someone who is bleeding profusely will be seen before another person with a broken toe.

Triage explains why some patients can sit in the waiting area for long periods of time without being seen by a physician, while others are taken in immediately. Everyone who comes to the emergency room feels ill and hates to be kept waiting, but remember, the triage principle protects you, as well. "First come, first served" would not be an ethical policy for the ER.

SOME REASONS NOT TO GO TO AN EMERGENCY ROOM

Your regular doctor is out of town.
You don't feel well in the middle of the night and you couldn't sleep anyway.
Chronic back pain.
Bad cold.
Need a checkup.
Ran out of pills.

Although triage may make waiting unavoidable, one way to decrease your waiting time is by visiting the ER when it is least busy. In general, from late afternoon to midnight is the ER's busiest time. The scene is one of bustling activity as doctors and nurses strain to get everyone taken care of. There are constant interruptions by sicker patients, telephone calls, and the occasional combative patient who needs to be restrained. If you are not deathly ill, avoid these times at all costs, for you may languish in the waiting room for hours. A mixed blessing is when the long wait results in a major elevation of your blood pressure to dangerous levels and catapults you to the front of the line.

After midnight and during the early morning and afternoon are generally quieter times in most emergency rooms. Most people tend to get sickest at night, so daytime hours are slower.

What kind of doctor will I see?

This depends on the type of hospital one goes to, and also in which state. In New York State, for example, emergency rooms must now be staffed by licensed physicians and supervised by board certified attending physicians so that there is always someone present with advanced training in patient care. While this improves the overall quality of the ER, some patients are miffed at another effect: Many private physicians feel less obligated to see their patients who are admitted to the ER, since they are confident that their patients will get good care.

Some rural hospitals may not have a physician present at all times. Nurses or physician assistants may not only do the initial triage, but also handle minor emergencies themselves without ever having a physician see the patient. Other hospital emergency rooms may be staffed by residents who are moonlighting to earn extra money. In a small suburban ER, for example, a young physician who has completed three years of internal-medicine training may be responsible for the care of every patient who comes into the ER. Five years after his last exposure to pediatrics and surgery, he diagnoses and treats children, and sutures some fairly serious cuts. There is backup available by phone if needed, but interestingly enough, it is rarely necessary.

What shall I bring to the ER with me?

Unless you are seriously ill or injured, bring something to do while waiting—a book to read, a sweater to knit, a crossword puzzle to complete.

A physician you are seeing for the first time will find it very helpful if you bring a current list of your medications and their dosages. It is also a good idea to keep a narrative list of your major illnesses and how they have been treated.

If you are a cardiac patient, always bring a copy of your last electrocardiogram with you to the emergency room. If you have any type of unusual history or abnormal finding on your physical examination, such as a heart murmur, make sure you know about it and are prepared to discuss it with another physician. This will save you a great deal of uncertainty and grief, because if you have an abnormality that is already known and evaluated, it *may* not need to be reevaluated.

Why is there sometimes a delay in transferring from the ER to a hospital room?

A frequent complaint voiced by emergency room patients and their families concerns timely transport to the patient floor. Even when a bed has been secured, it can seem an interminable wait until one finally leaves the chaos of the ER. One patient muttered, "What are they doing upstairs? Having a party while I wait?"

There are several reasons for delays. After a patient has been discharged from a hospital bed, all the linens must be changed, the room cleaned and disinfected, and all perishable equipment replaced. This takes time.

Additionally, patients are generally not brought to a new room during change of shift. Nurses and aides work in eight- to twelve-hour shifts, and when one group leaves to go home and another group arrives, the departing group must pass on all the important information about the patients to the new group. Obviously, without the sharing of knowledge, nobody would know what had transpired over the past shift. Understandably, nurses prefer not to be interrupted during this changeover. Accepting a new patient on the floor is very time-consuming and can wait until change of shift is over.

Who gets admitted to the hospital?

Every hospital has its own system for determining which emergency room patients qualify for admission. When the hospital is empty, patients are admitted who may not be all that sick. When all the beds are full, even very ill patients may not be admitted, but referred for next-day follow-up by their private physicians or clinic.

Each service, or department, also has its own method of determining whether admitted patients go to the intensive care unit or to a regular bed. This assignment, too, is dependent on bed availability on the various patient floors. If intensive care units are almost full, the last beds are reserved for major emergencies. If the units are sparsely populated, patients may be admitted there for simple observation.

What if there are no available beds in the hospital?

This happens quite frequently at university hospitals nowadays. In an effort to stay solvent, hospitals must be full at all times. Just as an empty hotel room generates no income, neither does an empty hospital bed. This means that there will be days when there are no available beds for emergency admissions. Two things then happen. Patients who are clearly sick enough to need hospitalization are parked overnight, frequently on a hospital gurney, in the emergency room. If the hospital takes emergency cases brought in by ambulance, it goes on "diversion"—all ambulances are told to take patients to another hospital. Not a happy situation if all your medical care has occurred in one specific hospital and you are forced to go somewhere else. But it is just part of the increasingly complicated challenges facing emergency rooms and the people who rely on them.

CHAPTER 9

FROM MORNING ROUNDS TO EVENING VISITORS: THE HOSPITAL DAY FOR TRADITIONAL ADMISSIONS

If you have a traditional admission, after you're through in the admissions office, a transport person escorts you to your room and deposits your chart at the nursing station. Until an intern or resident comes to greet and examine you, you have a while to look around your new "home." (See Chapter 4, "Planning and Preparing for Surgery," for a comparison of traditional, same-day, and ambulatory admissions.)

YOUR HOSPITAL ROOM

The standard hospital room is semiprivate—but not all semiprivate rooms are created equal. In most new community hospitals, a semiprivate room is a large, clean, bright space, with a private bathroom and shower that you share with only one other patient. But in an old university hospital in a large city, a semiprivate room is often small and may be shared by three or more people, and the bathroom is down the hall.

Decor is minimal: Besides a bed, you'll have a lamp, a nightstand, a bedstand for your meal trays, and perhaps a free-standing locker for your clothing. A curtain can be pulled around the bed for privacy. Fairly simple, but functional.

Upgrading to a private room is expensive. Few insurance plans pay for the cost of a private room. In a university hospital, the daily cost of a private room may be $500 to $750 more than what your insurance covers for a semiprivate room. Even if you want to splurge, a private room may not be available, since these rooms are often used as isolation units for patients with communicable diseases.

You can, however, maintain a degree of privacy in a semiprivate room. You have the right to insist on maintaining privacy during examinations and tests, regardless of who is performing them. No one is so busy or so important that the simple courtesy of pulling a curtain should be forgotten. Unfortunately, sometimes it is inadvertently overlooked and the offender must be reminded.

It is not only important for you and your roommate(s) to respect each other's privacy, but also for you to insist that your visitors do so as well. Be aware that if your roommate and his or her visitors are intolerable, you have the right to demand a change of room.

THE DAILY ROUTINE

At some point after you unpack and change out of your clothes, a nurse, medical student, intern, resident, and/or consulting physician will come in to take a history and examine you. (See Chapter 11, "The Hospital Chart.")

What happens next depends on how sick you feel. If you are quite ill or in pain, you should and will be expedited through your tests, X rays, consultations, and exams. If your condition is less serious, you may have quite a bit of time on your hands until your own tests and exams are done.

You may feel overwhelmed and tired by the exams, questions, and tests, but they are all done with one end in sight: to know you inside out so that you can leave the hospital healthier than you came in. The Latin phrase *res ipse locquitur* (the facts speak for themselves) applies. The system works.

REVEILLE

In the hospital, people really do wake you up at the crack of dawn. In order for the nursing and medical staff to get everything done in a timely fashion, the day has to start early. But it's unlikely that you slept that well anyway. Did it seem that every time you were about to fall asleep, somebody came in to check on you? It would be worse if no-body came in, wouldn't it?

The first thing the nurse does is check your vital signs. If you're having surgery, you'll wait to be prepped and taken to the operating room (see Chapter 17, "The Operating Room"). If you're not having surgery, then just when you are about to fall back to sleep, the house staff arrives. You are examined and any dressings are changed. Once they leave, you think it is finally time for a short nap. Wrong! Just as your eyes are about to close, the attending physician or surgeon arrives.

What follows depends on your condition and why you have been hospitalized. Incapacitated patients are bathed, fed, and have their linens changed. Patients who are less ill are guided through their morning ablutions or left alone to wash up at their own speed.

Sometime before breakfast, the blood-drawing technician usually arrives. Blood drawing and intravenous technicians are generally very good at what they do. They do the same thing over and over again, literally hundreds of times in a week, so having your blood taken or an IV placed should be relatively painless and rapid.

Unless you're having surgery, breakfast is next on the agenda, and you are probably finished eating by nine o'clock.

CAVEAT

If you are having surgery and you are given a meal tray, do not eat; if you do, your surgery will have to be canceled.

If you have not been scheduled for a major procedure, the day is generally filled with hours of boredom, intermittently interrupted by testing or treatment, and punctuated, of course, by morning rounds.

MORNING ROUNDS

After interns, residents, and fellows (or house-staff team) come into your room by ones and twos to interrupt your fitful sleep, eight or nine people converge in your room in a long-standing hospital tradition called morning rounds. This A.M. perambulation serves many functions: It guides patient care and planning, enhances safety, and fulfills a vital teaching function for the house staff. Rounds enable all the doctors on the team to speak with the patients and review laboratory data each morning. (See Chapter 14, "Your Hospital Team.")

Generally, rounds include an examination of the patients by the intern and resident assigned to them, as well as by the on-call intern. The examination is usually cursory and limited to the patient's main problem and any unresolved issues that need to be addressed during the day. For example, if a patient admitted with an acute myocardial infarction (MI), or heart attack, develops gout, the doctors will examine the affected joint and the heart. If there are any unusual findings, some of the rest of the team may want to examine the patient, too.

You always have the right to limit the exams and to insist on privacy. But be aware that by doing so, you may be depriving yourself of some potentially valuable input. The exchange of ideas during rounds works to the patient's advantage. It is not only the most senior physician on rounds who exhibits great insights and makes dazzling suggestions regarding a patient's care. The entire team is encouraged to offer and discuss ideas.

Group rounds contribute to patient safety. In this day and age, most interns and residents no longer spend every night or every other night in the hospital; they are "on-call" (present in the hospital) only every three or four nights. To a large extent, the modified schedule has been mandated by local and state governments in a misguided attempt to improve patient care. Reasoning that tired interns or residents are more apt to make a mistake, legislators failed to realize that this means that two out of every three nights on surgical services and three out of every four nights on medical services the resident physician directly responsible for your care is not available.

Rounds, therefore, allow the other members of your team to be familiar with your case in the event of a sudden, life-threatening emergency in the middle of the night. Dr. A, racing to see Dr. B's patient, does not have to stop first at the nurses' station and read the chart in order to become familiar with the patient's situation; Dr. A remembers the patient from the morning rounds.

Final decisions are made by the patient's attending physician, frequently after consulting with the house staff. If you have any questions, ask your attending, rather than house, officers, who may not always have the information and experience to answer questions.

HIERARCHY

When in doubt about where in the doctor hierarchy someone fits, a good first guide is to look at the length of the white coat and the color of the pants or skirt. In general, there are only two lengths of coat; the longer the coat, the higher in the hierarchy the doctor is. In addition, medical students and interns generally wear white pants and/or skirts because they are supplied and cleaned by the hospital and it makes them feel more like a real doctor. Few, if any, residents or attending physicians wear them.

TESTS

Most tests (except blood tests) are not performed in your room. An escort picks you up and takes you to the site of the testing, either by wheelchair or stretcher. This sounds simple, but can be one of the most frustrating aspects of a hospitalization. Imagine being left in a cold hallway, strapped to a stretcher, and having to go to the bathroom. The passage of time in this circumstance gives painful new meaning to the term *slow motion*.

When you go for a test, take a friend, if possible, and/or a book, a magazine, or a small radio or tape player with headphones. Wear slippers and a robe over your hospital gown so you won't be cold. Also, if you are larger than average size, you may find that the hospital gown doesn't fit. To preserve your modesty, ask for two gowns and put one on backward so you have full coverage, front and back.

EVENING HOURS

Dinner is over. Visitors have left. Boredom intensifies. This is "good boredom," because if you are getting lots of attention at this time of night, it must mean that you are really sick. Even if you are antitelevision, order one when you get to the hospital. Many times, you just cannot concentrate enough to curl up with *Crime and Punishment* or even a less-challenging tome. If there was ever a time for which television was made to order, evenings in the hospital is it.

VISITING HOURS

Every hospital has its own policy regarding visiting hours. Some hospitals allow children to visit, while others require all visitors to be over ten years old. Some hospitals permit extended visits, while others want guests in and out within an hour. Visitor policies can even vary floor by floor and unit by unit in the same hospital. However, some general principles apply:

- Visitors should be limited to only two or three at a time.
- In intensive care units, visits are generally limited to fifteen minutes at a time.
- Visiting hours are almost always late afternoon and early evening, and generally last until eight or nine o'clock.
- Children under a particular age are usually not permitted admission to any of the hospital floors. However, maternity floors may allow siblings of newborns to visit.

The wisdom behind the rules is that visitors should not tire patients or annoy their roommates. Although many hospitals are somewhat lax about strictly enforcing these rules, they really should be respected for the good of the patients. Let your friends and relatives know ahead of time whether you wish to have visitors. Be honest. You may find it helpful to delegate one person to "screen" your visitors and let people know if and when it is convenient for them to come. (See Chapter 20, "The Intensive Care Unit," for information on ICU visitors.)

SAFETY IN THE HOSPITAL

A hospital is a dynamic community with round-the-clock arrivals, departures, and activity. And as a community, a hospital has many of the problems—such as crime—that are associated with whatever larger community it belongs to. Both patients and their visitors need to use common sense and follow the same precautions they would as tourists in a new city.

Don't go into deserted or unlighted areas, either inside or outside the hospital.

Leave your valuables at home, or make sure they are not left unattended. Some hospitals have lockers or a safe for patients' valuables.

If you are lost, ask someone in a uniform for directions.

At night, park in lighted areas or a guarded garage.

CHAPTER 10

HOSPITAL FOOD

Mealtimes not only provide nourishment; they break up the hospital routine and give patients something to look forward to. Yet, eager anticipation often turns to disgruntled disappointment when hospital food fails to live up to the menu's promises. There can be a startling contrast between the menu's mouthwatering descriptions ("tender roast chicken with cornbread stuffing and fresh vegetable *garni*"), and the food that actually appears on the tray (a pallid drumstick with tasteless "stuffing" and a few limp green beans).

Sometimes the "food chain" goes *completely* awry; when the kitchen runs out of certain dishes or a food-service worker makes a mistake, the meal you receive may bear no resemblance to what you ordered. Anticipating mealtime takes on a whole new meaning: If you order "Chicken Surprise," you may feel surprised to receive any chicken at all!

Although people often joke about hospital food, the topic is actually a serious one. If meals are not appetizing, then you may not eat all you should to keep your strength up; if the tray you receive does not contain what you or your doctor ordered, then you may be eating food that is inappropriate for your condition.

Some hospitals have taken steps to salvage hospital food's reputation. They use more fresh vegetables and whole grains; they enable some patients to order meals from local restaurants; and they invite (and respond to) patient feedback on the quality of the food and presentation.

How Your Doctor Orders Your Meals

All hospital patients have a specific diet ordered for them by their responsible attending physician, who aims to match their diet and caloric intake to their particular medical situation. This can range from NPO (*non per os*, meaning "nothing by mouth") to a high-calorie, high-fat extravaganza. Since mistakes occasionally occur, always check your tray to make sure that you received the right one and to avoid eating foods that are not appropriate for your condition.

The typical IV bag. Most patients can be adequately nourished by a combination of intravenous fluids and oral intake. Most intravenous fluids are clear and contain dextrose, a simple sugar that the body converts to glucose and uses for energy; dextrose usually supplies several hundred calories a day. Dextrose in too high a concentration can be irritating to veins, so there are limits to how much can be delivered in a twenty-four-hour period.

Intravenous solutions may contain varying amounts of necessary minerals and vitamins, depending on the patient's needs. Because these needs may change fairly often (for example, patients with a high fever require much more intravenous fluid because they lose a great deal through skin evaporation), doctors and nurses review the directions for fluid administration on a daily basis.

High calories for postsurgical healing. A person who has recently undergone major surgery is generally in a catabolic state: The body is trying to repair itself by breaking down available sources of energy for immediate use. The healing process requires as many calories as possible, sometimes over three thousand calories per day. These calories may be taken by mouth, either in liquid or solid form, or supplied intravenously for those patients who cannot or will not eat.

Correcting nutritional deficits. Some people are so undernourished that a special intravenous catheter is inserted into a large vein to administer a high-fat and caloric liquid called a hyperalimentation diet. Unlike most intravenous solutions, which are clear, the fluids administered in a hyperalimentation diet are generally milky in appearance, because they are so high in fat.

Doctors often call upon a consultant, generally a surgeon, to devise the components of the diet, to place the central line, and to monitor its care in order to prevent any possible infection. It is always important for intravenous lines to be sterile, but hyperalimentation IVs require even stricter monitoring than typical IV lines because these highly caloric fluids tend to attract the growth of germs that can be very harmful if they enter the vascular system (veins and arteries) directly.

Liquid diets by mouth. Clear-liquid diets are ordered to cleanse the bowels prior to abdominal surgery, and for patients who are just beginning to eat again after major bowel surgery. Clear liquids (those you can see through, such as broth, gelatin, and juices) are easy to digest and don't require the bowels to work too hard. Full liquid diets may include soups, ice cream, and custards. They are the next step up for recovering patients as they progress toward a normal diet.

HOSPITAL FOOD ALTERNATIVES

Visitors may wish to bring you food, but remember to check with your doctor or nurse before consuming it, since it may conflict with your prescribed diet. If your doctor permits you to replace or supplement hospital food, check your hospital's policy on the availability of small, portable refrigerators.

If you have special needs, such as allergies or the desire for kosher or vegetarian meals, or want advice on planning your posthospital diet, ask to speak with the dietician. He or she can advise you about how to lower your intake of cholesterol, fat, or sugar; how to adjust calories in order to gain or lose weight; or how to alter your diet in response to certain medical conditions (e.g., patients with diverticulosis should avoid nuts, seeds, and certain other foods).

No one should choose a hospital on the basis of its food, but hospital administrators do want you to feel satisfied with your overall hospital experience. If you are unhappy with the food you receive, speak up and give the hospital a chance to make improvements.

BREAKFAST
Please circle your selections

DAY: M Tu W Th F Sa Su

Juices & Fruits

Orange Juice	Grapefruit Juice	Banana
Apple Juice	Prune Juice	Applesauce
Cranberry Juice	Stewed Prunes	Raisins

Cereals (please select Milk)

All Bran	Corn Flakes	Rice Krispies
Raisin Bran	Total	Oatmeal
Cheerios	Shredded Wheat	Cream of Wheat

Entrées & Accompaniments (choose 1)

Omelette: Plain Cheese Mushroom Spanish
Low Fat Omelette: Plain Cheese Mushroom Spanish
French Toast Home-Fried Potatoes
Buttermilk Pancakes Sausage Patties
Maple-Flavored Syrup Unsweetened Maple-Flavored Syrup Catsup

Side Orders

Plain Yogurt	Swiss Cheese	Cottage Cheese
Fruit Yogurt	Monterey Jack Cheese	Hard Cooked Egg
	Cheddar Cheese	

Breads & Spreads

Bagel:	Muffin:	Margarine	Fruit Spread
Plain	Blueberry	Butter	Cream Cheese
Cinnamon Raisin	Corn	Jelly	Peanut Butter
Whole Wheat	Bran		

Condiments & Beverages

Extra Sugar	Skim Milk	Coffee
Sugar Substitute	2% Milk	Decaf Coffee
Creamer	Whole Milk	Tea/Lemon
Vanilla Milkshake	Chocolate Milkshake	Herbal Tea/Lemon
		Cocoa

Guest _____ Location _____

Diet: GENERAL (Blue Condiment Kit)

LUNCH
Please circle your selections

DAY: M Tu W Th F Sa Su   LF = Low Fat

Appetizers
Apple Juice Grape Juice   Vegetable Soup   Chicken Orzo Soup
Fruit Punch Cranberry Juice   Soup of the Day Cream Soup of the Day

Entrées (Choose 1)
Grilled Beefsteak Patty   Macaroni & Cheese
Herbed Chicken Breast   Gourmet Beef Stew
Pizza   Pasta with Meat Sauce
Roast Loin of Pork   **Chef's Special**   See reverse

Cold Plates:
  Tuna Salad   Grilled Chicken   Cottage Cheese & Fruit

Sandwiches: *whole wheat or white (circle one)*
  Turkey   Swiss Cheese
  Tuna Salad   Peanut Butter & Jelly
  Ham & American Cheese

Salads, Dressings & Accompaniments
Garden Fresh Salad   Dressing: French   LF French
Carrot & Celery Sticks   Parmesan Cheese   Sour Cream
Coleslaw   Catsup   Dijon Mustard
Green Bean Vinaigrette   Mayonnaise   Cranberry Sauce

Breads & Spreads
7-Grain Roll   Crackers   Margarine
Dinner Roll   Pretzels   Butter

Dessert Cart (Choose only 1)
Fresh Fruit   Apple Pie   Sugar Cookies
Applesauce   Chocolate Cake   Vanilla Pudding
Fruit Yogurt   Angel Food Cake   Chocolate Pudding

Condiments & Beverages
Extra Sugar   Skim Milk   Coffee
Sugar Substitute   2% Milk   Decaf Coffee
Creamer   Whole Milk   Tea/Lemon
Vanilla Milkshake   Chocolate Milkshake Herbal Tea/Lemon

Guest _____   Location _____

Diet: GENERAL (Blue Condiment Kit)

DINNER
Please circle your selections

DAY: M Tu W Th F Sa Su   LF = Low Fat

Appetizers.
Apple Juice   Grape Juice   Vegetable Soup   Chicken Orzo Soup
Fruit Punch   Cranberry Juice   Soup of the Day   Cream Soup of the Day

Entrées (Choose 1)
Roast Turkey   Chicken with Mushroom & Wine Sauce
Meatloaf   Lasagna
Poached Salmon   Vegetarian Chili
Pot Roast   **Chef's Special**

Cold Plates:
   Tuna Salad   Grilled Chicken   Cottage Cheese & Fruit

Sandwiches: *whole wheat or white (circle one)*
   Turkey   Swiss Cheese
   Tuna Salad   Peanut Butter & Jelly
   Ham & American Cheese

Salads, Dressings & Accompaniments
Garden Fresh Salad   Dressing: Italian   LF Italian
Carrot & Celery Sticks   Parmesan Cheese   Sour Cream
Coleslaw   Catsup   Dijon Mustard
Green Bean Vinaigrette   Mayonnaise   Cranberry Sauce

Breads & Spreads
7-Grain Roll   Crackers   Margarine
Dinner Roll   Pretzels   Butter

Dessert Cart (Choose only 1)
Fresh Fruit   Apple Pie   Sugar Cookies
Applesauce   Chocolate Cake   Vanilla Pudding
Fruit Yogurt   Angel Food Cake   Chocolate Pudding

Condiments & Beverages
Extra Sugar   Skim Milk   Coffee
Sugar Substitute   2% Milk   Decaf Coffee
Creamer   Whole Milk   Tea/Lemon
Vanilla Milkshake   Chocolate Milkshake   Herbal Tea/Lemon

Guest _____   Location _____

Diet: GENERAL (Blue Condiment Kit)

CHAPTER 11

THE HOSPITAL CHART

The hospital chart is like a diary, a confidential record of every day of your hospital stay. Your doctors and other medical professionals write everything from their impressions of your progress, or lack thereof, to the details of your mental state and the state of your bowels. Years ago, doctors occasionally wrote amusing notes and idle speculations in chart notes, but now, because of potential litigation, the prose tends to be dry and minimal. The hands of lawyers are found everywhere in medicine.

> **THE ADMISSION HISTORY AND PHYSICAL EXAM**
>
> **Chief complaint**
> **History of present illness**
> **Past medical history**
> **Social history**
> **Family history**
> **Review of systems**
> **Physical examination**
> **Impression**
> **Plan**

The initial section of the chart contains the information you gave when interviewed by the attending physicians, residents, interns, nurses, and medical students responsible for your care. The rest of the chart includes lab results, medical notes, and previous hospital records.

TAKING A HISTORY

Your history is taken and a physical exam is done when you arrive in your hospital room (although, if you are an emergency admission, a brief history may have been taken in the emergency room).

Interviews and physical exams may be done by an intern, resident, medical student, nurse practitioner, or physician's assistant. You may find that you are interviewed by more than one person, often by the least experienced first, and that you are asked questions you have already answered. Try not to get frustrated. The more they know you inside out (literally and figuratively), the better your care will be. And being interviewed by more than one person is a kind of checks-and-balance system; one may ask a question that someone else didn't think of, or you may give slightly different answers to similar questions, indicating the need to clarify information.

Some questions may seem embarrassing, such as inquiries into your sex life, your emotional frame of mind, your bathroom habits, or your use of alcohol or other drugs. It's important to answer all questions honestly, for the answers are significant to your care. All information is kept confidential, and will not be disclosed to your employer, family, or anyone else without your permission.

The components of a patient's history have not changed in fifty years, but the order in which they are recorded in the chart may vary from hospital to hospital. What follows are the components of a complete history and physical examination, as they would be done at a university hospital.

THE CHIEF COMPLAINT

Most admission histories begin with a one- or two-line statement, usually in the patient's own words, on why he or she has come to the hospital. The chief complaint is meant to focus a reader's attention on the main problem, but every medical professional knows that it is no substitute for the detailed history that follows.

HISTORY OF THE PRESENT ILLNESS

The History of the Present Illness (HPI) is a narrative description of the problem that has brought the patient to the hospital, and some of the factors that have contributed directly to the present problem. For example, the HPI for a patient admitted for angina (heart pain) will have a discussion of their smoking habits, but not of a previous skin cancer. For trainees in medicine, learning what to include and exclude is learning medicine itself.

The HPI, and much of the rest of the chart, is written in a series of abbreviations. For example, if Joseph Johnson is a fifty-nine-year-old white male, with a twenty-five-year history of smoking three packs of cigarettes a day, the chart will read: "JJ is a 59 yo W♂ c̄ a 25 yr HX of smoking 3 PPD."

PAST MEDICAL HISTORY (PMHx)

"Past medical history" includes reports on previous surgeries and hospitalizations, other serious illnesses, medications taken, allergies, and habits (smoking, alcohol consumption, etc.).

SOCIAL HISTORY

"Social history" recounts your marital status, occupation, and living situation (home, skilled nursing facility, etc.).

FAMILY HISTORY

This section includes the ages and health problems of your parents, siblings, children, and other close relatives. An attempt is always made to discover the presence of a familial problem. For example, if you are admitted with a cough and fever, it would be important to state that your father had tuberculosis during World War II. Tuberculosis can be transmitted at any age and lay dormant for many years. Knowing that TB was present in your family might lead your physician to the correct diagnosis sooner.

REVIEW OF SYSTEMS

"Review of systems" can be an exhaustive, lengthy series of questions regarding the function of every organ system in the body. Medical students often ask lists of questions and write down every response, an approach intended to familiarize them with all of the organ systems and their problems. More seasoned physicians tend to explore in depth those aspects that are crucial in the present situation, and only touch on other aspects of health. They are sensitive to time constraints, and are experienced enough to know which information is tangential and which is truly relevant.

Let's say that you are admitted for the repair of a hernia. An attending physician who comes to see you might ask only one question about each organ system, such as, "Have you had any problems with your lungs?" A medical student, on the other hand, might ask, "Have you had any trouble breathing? Have you been coughing lately? Have you coughed up blood? Are you short of breath? Does it hurt when you take a deep breath? Do you wake up short of breath in the middle of the night?" The list can seem endless when applied to every organ system in the body.

THE PHYSICAL EXAMINATION

The physical examination begins with a description of the patient's general appearance, age, gender, and perhaps ethnic background. The vital signs are next, and include temperature, pulse rate, blood pressure, and respiratory rate (how many times per minute the patient breathes). A description of the examination of the patient's organ systems follows, with special attention to any abnormal findings. There are four components of any description of an organ system: inspection, palpation, percussion, and auscultation.

Inspection. Doctors are trained to inspect people in a scientific way. For example, they observe the patient's overall skin tone: Is it jaundiced, pale, cyanotic (blue from lack of oxygen), or flushed from exertion? They also assess the skin's turgor, or firmness, which indicates whether the person has enough body fluids (Is the skin overly dry?) and state of cleanliness: Is the patient bathed and well-groomed? Are nails clean and trimmed? Is the patient unkempt, soiled, or apparently incontinent? These and other factors may all be relevant to a patient's overall problem. For example, a disheveled, soiled appearance may not be directly related to a person's pneumonia, but may suggest alcohol abuse, which indicates the need to check for a specific type of bacteria that may be more serious than an ordinary pneumonia.

Palpation. The laying on of hands. In our society, the right to touch strangers in private places is given only to physicians, nurses, and other caregivers. This is an important trust, and medical professionals are taught early on to divorce themselves from any prurient interest. A good physical examination includes the palpation of every area and organ in the body—the skin, hair, glands, breasts, heart, liver, spleen, abdomen, reproductive organs, and so on.

Percussion. The term that describes what physicians do when they tap their fingers on you. Like musical instruments, the various parts of the body make different sounds when percussed. These differences can offer clues to the state of health. For example, normal, air-filled lungs sound hollow. But when there is fluid around a lung (a pleural effusion), the sound is deadened. A chest X ray is not always needed to make a diagnosis.

Auscultation. Listening, generally through a stethoscope, is auscultation. Different organs of the body make different sounds when they are healthy or diseased. For example, normal heart sounds are *lub-dub, lub-dub*. When a heart valve is damaged, you hear *lub-whoosh-dub*. Normal lungs sound like a breeze when air flows through them. But when a person has pneumonia, during inhalation there are sounds like crackling paper. These are known as rales.

THE CLINICAL IMPRESSION

So far, the history and physical exam have consisted of assembling facts. When both have been completed, it is time for the physician to speculate about the exact nature of your problem. Your physician's theory of what is wrong with you is noted as the clinical impression.

WHO GIVES PHYSICAL EXAMS?

Nurse practitioners
Medical students
Interns
Residents
Fellows
Attending physicians

THE PLAN

The plan is a list of the examinations required for a correct diagnosis, or a discussion of the proposed treatment. For example, if the clinical impression is pneumonia, the plan might include a chest X ray, arterial blood gases to measure the lungs' ability to absorb oxygen, oxygen by mask if needed, intravenous fluids, antibiotics, and respiratory therapy to help the patient cough.

CHART UPKEEP, RULES, AND STORAGE

THE REMAINDER OF THE CHART

In addition to the admission history and physical exam, the chart includes notes on the patient's condition and progress. Notes are entered at least once a day. Patients who are unstable or receiving new treatments several times a day may have several notes over the course of the day. Progress notes address the events of the day, the results of important tests, and recommendations by attending physicians, consultants, physical therapists, and others.

Chart notes are not all created equal. Some are incomprehensible due to the infamous penmanship problems of doctors. Some notes add nothing new, but are jotted down just to indicate that a doctor was there and saw the patient. Nevertheless, overall, the chart is crucial— the only way for all pertinent information to be shared, since the care providers are rarely all present on the patient floor at the same time.

CHART RULES AND REGULATIONS

A hospital chart is a legal record. Hospitals have reams of rules on how to write in it, what is appropriate to include, how to sign progress notes, even how to correct a penmanship mistake. Notes are supposed to be written in black or blue ink so that they are legible when photocopied, except for procedure notes (such as a spinal tap), which are written in red ink.

STORAGE OF MEDICAL RECORDS

Once a patient is discharged from the hospital, the chart is sent to the medical records department for storage. It is collated and its components are bound together. If an official written report on a hospitalization is not available until after discharge, it will be added in the record room.

Old charts are never discarded. In the event that you are hospitalized again, old charts are always helpful. They contain information that you may have forgotten, EKGs that can be retrieved and compared with the present ones to see if a change has occurred, as well as a host of other information. Because of space considerations, charts more than two or three years old may be stored in an out-of-hospital facility or put on microfilm. (In contrast, physicians in private practice need to keep records for only six and a half years, or until the patient is twenty-one years old, whichever comes later.) This makes charts harder to retrieve in a timely fashion, but no hospital has the space to store the massive number of charts that accumulate over the years.

COMMON CHART ABBREVIATIONS

W = white   ♂ = man   C̀ = with
B = black   ♀ = woman   S̀ = without
H = Hispanic

ABG   = arterial blood gases
AML   = acute myelogenous leukemia
ASHD = arteriosclerotic heart disease
CAD   = coronary artery disease
CML   = chronic myelogenous leukemia
CP   = chest pain
CXR   = chest X ray
EKG   = electrocardiogram (the K is derived from the German spelling)
HCT   = hematocrit
HG   = hemoglobin
HX   = history
IEP   = immunoelectrophoresis
Ig   = immunoglobulin
LMD   = local medical doctor
MI   = myocardial infarction (heart attack)
PFT   = pulmonary function test
PID   = pelvic inflammatory disease
PPD   = purified protein derivative used as a skin test for TB
PPD or PACK/DAY = packs per day (refers to cigarettes)
PMHx = past medical history
PVD   = peripheral vascular disease
RBC   = red blood cells
RX   = therapy or treatment
SIEP = serum immunoelectrophoresis
SX   = symptoms
TAH   = total abdominal hysterectomy
TB   = tuberculosis
TFT   = thyroid function tests
TURP = transurethral prostatectomy
TX   = transfusion
UGI   = upper gastrointestinal
URI   = upper respiratory illness
UTI   = urinary tract infection
WBC   = white blood cells

CC: 75 yo ♂ c̄ 3 hr. of chest pain, "Like an elephant sitting on my chest."

HPI: 1st NYH admission for this 75 yo ♂ c̄ a HX 50 pack years smoking, ↑ cholesterol, bad FHx, gout, HTN and known PVD: well controlled until 3 hr. ago when he developed severe 8/10 mid-chest pain radiating to his L arm and associated c̄ dyspnea, sweating and palpitations. 1 hr ago, took a 2 yr. old nitroglycerin under his tongue → no relief → called 911 and presented to ER.

FHx: Father died at 68 of MI

Mother died at 90 "natural causes"

1 brother had triple CABG

SHx: Works as a fireman

Married, 3 children

ETOH: 3–4 beers/day

Drugs: ō

PMHx: Surgery - Gallbladder removal 1984

Appendectomy 1950

Allergies - PCN → rash

Meds   - Aspirin 324 mg 8 AM

Isordil 10 mg TID

Norvasc 5 mg 8 AM

ROS: Neuro - rare dizzy spells

Skin - ō

HEENT cataract L eye

Lungs - mild dyspnea on exertion

CVS - see HPI

GI   - nl bowels

GU   - gets up 2X at night to urinate sexual function ↓

PE: 160/90 PR 66 RR 12 Afib

HEENT: normocephalic, L cataract

Lungs: clear to A + P

COR: $S_1 S_2$ nl 1/6 SEM → carotids
no gallops, clicks

Abdomen: $\bar{o}$ masses or tenderness

Rectal: nl prostate $\bar{o}$ masses

Ext: 1+ pulses, $\bar{o}$ edema

Neuro: Oriented X3
Reflexes 2+
Strength 5/5

Labs: EKG   - NSR at 80
ST elevation II, III, AVF
CXR   - nl

$$\frac{140 \mid 3.8}{98 \mid 24} \quad \text{BUN 14 Glucose 114} \quad \text{CR 1.0}$$

HG 14/Hct 42/WBC 9600/PHS 420,000

Imp: 75 yo ♂ $\bar{o}$ multiple cardiac risk factors and EKG evidence of acute MI

Plan: Admit to CCV
TPA given in ER
Nitropaste 1" q 4 hr.
Heparin to keep PTT at 80
Cardiac enzymes X3
O_2 by nasal canula

CHAPTER 12

THE NURSES

Nurses are dedicated, trained, professional women and men who devote their lives to the care of the sick. They are the crucial point of contact between patients and doctors, patients and procedures, patients and treatment. Above all, they function in an atmosphere of potential life-or-death decision-making on a daily basis. Even when all seems calm and they are joking at the nursing station, an emergency can shatter that calm in an instant.

Because nurses are the most visible and accessible members of the hospital staff, they get more firsthand feedback from patients than anyone else. The feedback can range from confiding, joking, and appreciation to tears, outrage, frustration, and attacks. Nurses understand that patients often need to "vent." But nurses are also human and have limits to their tolerance.

One important nursing function is to translate "doctorspeak" into English. For example, during rounds, a doctor may tell a patient that he'll have a "sono" that afternoon. Later, the nurse translates: *Sono* is an abbreviation for sonography, a sound-wave test of the abdomen. It doesn't hurt, and it doesn't involve radiation.

TYPES OF NURSES

Like physicians, nurses have various types of degrees and titles, all representing different levels of training.

Licensed Practical Nurse (LPN). With two years of nursing training following high school, LPNs may take blood pressure and temperature and administer medication, but may not give narcotics. The clinical responsibility of an LPN is the most restricted of any of the degree nurses; they must work at all times under the direct clinical supervision of a physician or registered nurse.

Registered Nurse (RN). She or he has either completed a three-year training program at a university-affiliated hospital, or received a bachelor's degree and an RN certificate from a four-year program. In either case, the training and roles are identical—but the potential for promotion and furthering of nursing education is dramatically different. A four-year-degree nurse can go on to get a master's degree and a doctorate, or may take further nursing courses in clinical specialties and become a nurse practitioner in pediatrics, primary care, obstetrics, anesthesia, etc. (see below). A three-year-degree nurse must first obtain the requisite college credits to achieve parity with a four-year nurse.

Nurse Practitioner. This nurse not only has a bachelor's degree in nursing but has received the equivalent of a master's degree. Nurse practitioners generally specialize in a particular aspect of primary care, and many states have passed or are considering legislation to allow them to function almost independently. This has created some friction with physicians as turf battles begin to break out. The nurses argue that they provide more humane, time-intensive treatment at lower cost. Physicians counter that since nurse practitioners have been trained by other nurses, they do not have the scientific underpinnings provided by four years of medical school to provide adequate medical care.

There's no question that many nurse practitioners are capable of going beyond the traditional nurse's role in such aspects of primary care as healthy baby care (routine checkups, immunizations, counseling) and the management of such problems as mild hypertension or mild diabetes. If a person has a single problem that needs frequent monitoring, extensive counseling, and minor medication adjustments, a nurse practitioner can almost certainly handle the case safely and inexpensively. However, more complex cases, such as multiple diagnoses or multiple organ system disease, should be handled by physicians. The

borderline between "mild" and "complex" cases, of course, is contro-
versial, and probably should be determined in part by the talents and experience of the individual caregivers. At the very least, however, people
with a significant medical condition should have an annual evaluation by
a physician even if they are followed by a nurse practitioner.

Physician's Assistant (PA or RPA). He or she is not a nurse, but
a college graduate who has completed an additional two and a half
years of training in an accredited PA program and passed a nationally
administered exam; PAs must be recertified every seven years. Their
training is provided by physicians, and in many cases, classes are shared
with medical students.

The number of physician's assistants has grown significantly, since
they can perform some of the same functions as a physician at a lower
cost. The major difference between them and doctors is that PAs are
not required to go to medical school or to do an internship or residency. They provide primary care under the supervision of a physician.
PAs can take medical histories, conduct physical examinations, draw
blood, do sutures, etc. More and more, they are entering into specialties such as plastic and reconstructive surgery, and orthopedic surgery,
where they provide care under the guidance of the specialty physicians.
By doing the day-to-day ordering of tests and writing of notes, they
free physicians to spend more time in the operating room. In some
states, physician's assistants may write prescriptions and even dispense
controlled substances (pain relievers, narcotics).

NURSES OF THE HOSPITAL STAFF

Regardless of their level of training, nurses who work on patient floors
often perform similar functions, such as delivering medications on
time, caring for intravenous lines, helping with the patients' daily hygiene, attending to surgical dressings, etc. Often, these non-MD professionals are a great resource for interns and residents because they
have done the same work for years, as opposed to a three-month rotation. Nurses often help young doctors recognize common problems,
understand hospital protocol, and generally get up-to-speed.

The nursing staff of each hospital floor may differ slightly, depending on the complexity of the patients' conditions. In an intensive care
unit (ICU), where there are very sick patients with many problems,
multiple intravenous lines, and the need for continuous monitoring,

---

THE NURSE'S BASIC RESPONSIBILITIES

Monitor and observe patients and inform the responsible physician of any changes in the patients' status.

Dispense medications and intravenous fluids as ordered by the physicians.

Care for all wounds, dressings, and lines as prescribed by the medical staff.

Coordinate and supervise other medical personnel, such as aides and therapists who are helping in patients' daily care and needs (e.g., personal hygiene, diet, therapy).

Educate patients about their care and medical needs.

Interact with patients and family members on a personal and emotional level to help them cope with a crisis situation.

---

there may be one nurse for every two patients. On a rehabilitation floor, where patients are recuperating and regaining strength, there may be two nurses for twenty-five patients.

Generally, three shifts of nurses cover a twenty-four-hour period; each shift is eight hours. There are always more nurses present during daylight hours when the lion's share of therapy and diagnostic tests are done. Each shift has one person in charge; the overall head nurse usually works during the day shift. The head nurse's main responsibilities are scheduling, troubleshooting, and teaching new nurses the ropes.

In order to assure continuity of care, so that each shift knows what occurred on the previous shift, there is a "sign out" process when there is only a skeleton staff caring for patient needs while the other nurses have conferences about their charges. Patients who try ringing for a nurse at this time can become very frustrated by the delay in responding.

PRIVATE-DUTY NURSES

An expensive but satisfying way to guarantee immediate access to a nurse is to hire a private-duty nurse—a nurse's aide, LPN, or RN. The private-duty nurse is responsible for caring for only the patient who hires her or him. The floor nursing staff are usually ecstatic to see "private duties," because it means there's one less patient who will require extensive care.

Upon arriving for work, private-duty nurses report to the head nurse and announce their presence. If they are RNs, they can do everything a floor nurse can do: bathe the patient, administer medications, monitor vital signs (blood pressure, pulse rate, breathing, temperature), and interact with the family. Unfortunately, only the most costly insurance plans cover private nurses, even if physicians feel they are necessary. In the final analysis, if you can afford a private nurse when you are quite ill, by all means, hire one. Ask the nurse on the floor how to find the hospital's private-duty nursing office.

Nurses are the backbone of the hospital. They are deeply involved in patients' minute-to-minute care, and provide patients and their families with meaningful emotional support and patient education. Nurses often have been taken for granted, but increasingly, these knowledgeable professionals are getting the respect and responsibility they deserve. Ironically, however, just as some doctors are edgy about having nurses "encroach" on their territory, nurses, too, are facing encroachment by nurses' aides, licensed practical nurses, and others, as cost-cutting hospital bureaucracies seek to deliver certain aspects of nursing care for less money. While many nurses' aides and LPNs are highly capable, they cannot substitute for nurses in many respects. At the same time, as nurses are given an expanding role in the medical care of patients who are not critically ill, one hopes that they will still have time to offer patients the support that has been a hallmark of traditional nursing care.

PATIENT HISTORY

NURSE'S CHART

UNIT:	DATE:	TIME:	AGE:

VITAL SIGNS	T	P	R	BP	HGT	WT

METHOD OF ADMISSION:
☐ WALKING   ☐ WHEELCHAIR   ☐ STRETCHER
☐ OTHER (SPECIFY):

IDENTIBAND PRESENT AND CORRECT: ☐ YES   ☐ NO

ACCOMPANIED BY (SPECIFY RELATIONSHIP):

STATED REASON FOR ADMISSION:

ADMITTING DIAGNOSIS/PROCEDURE:

OTHER ILLNESSES/PRIOR HOSPITALIZATIONS:

ALLERGIES:

Self Care

SENSORY DEFICITS: ☐ NONE
☐ VISUALLY IMPAIRED   ☐ BLIND   ☐ HEARING IMPAIRED
☐ DEAF
☐ OTHER (SPECIFY)

ASSISTIVE DEVICES: ☐ NONE
USES   USES

☐ UPPER DENTURES	☐ WITH PT
☐ LOWER DENTURES	☐ WITH PT
☐ EYEGLASSES	☐ WITH PT
☐ CONTACT LENSES	☐ WITH PT
☐ HEARING AID	☐ WITH PT
☐ CANE	☐ WITH PT
☐ CRUTCHES	☐ WITH PT
☐ WALKER	☐ WITH PT
☐ PROSTHETIC DEVICE (specify)	☐ WITH PT
☐ OTHER (specify)	☐ WITH PT

ACTIVITIES REQUIRING ASSITANCE: ☐ NONE
☐ BATHING   ☐ TOILETING   ☐ EATING   ☐ AMBULATING
☐ DRESSING   ☐ MOVING TO AND FROM BED/CHAIR

CUSTOMARY DIET:

BOWEL HABITS:

BLADDER FUNCTION:

SLEEPING PATTERN:

Medications ☐ NONE
NAME, DOSE, FREQUENCY   # TIMES TAKEN TODAY

DISPOSITION OF MEDICATIONS BROUGHT TO HOSPITAL:
☐ NONE BROUGHT TO HOSPITAL
☐ GIVEN TO FAMILY/SIGNIFICANT OTHER
☐ OTHER (specify):

Indwelling Treatment Devices   ☐ NONE
☐ BROVIAC/HICKMAN   ☐ PERCUTANEOUS FEEDING
  CATHETER   TUBE
☐ PCA RELATED   ☐ HEPLOCK/PERIPHERAL IV
☐ PERITONEAL CATHETER   ☐ OTHER (SPECIFY):
☐ IMPLANTABLE VASCULAR
  ACCESS DEVICE

Social History

LIVES WITH:

DWELLING:

AGENCY/HOME CARE SUPPORT:

OCCUPATION:

LANGUAGE: ☐ ENGLISH   ☐ OTHER (SPECIFY):

ALCOHOL/DRUG USE:

SMOKING HISTORY:

DISPOSITION OF VALUABLES: ☐ PATIENT DENIES HAVING

ORIENTED TO UNIT (CHECK ALL THAT APPLY):
☐ CARE OF VALUABLES   ☐ BED CONTROLS
☐ VISITING HOURS   ☐ CALL LIGHT
☐ LOCATION OF BATHROOMS ☐ PHONE
☐ MEAL SERVICE   ☐ TV RENTAL
☐ SMOKE-FREE POLICY

MD NOTIFIED: (NAME)

NOTIFIED AT: _____ AM _____ PM

NURSE'S SIGNATURE/TITLE:

PRINT NAME:

NURSING ADMISSION ASSESSMENT

EDUCATIONAL ASSESSMENT

CHECK EACH ITEM (✔) OR MARK WITH AN ASTERISK (*). EXPLAIN ANY ASTERISK BELOW. CONSIDER HEALTH TEACHING NEEDS RELATED TO BREAST EXAMINATION, PAP SMEAR, TESTICULAR SELF-EXAMINATION, MENOPAUSE, SAFE SEX, ALCHOHOL AND DRUG USE, ETC.

☐ PT/S.O. UNDERSTANDS DIAGNOSIS AND REASON FOR HOSPITALIZATION
☐ PT/S.O. UNDERSTANDS MEDICATIONS OR DOES NOT TAKE MEDICATIONS

ASSESSMENT/**OTHER SIGNIFICANT FINDINGS**

FALL RISK ASSESSMENT

CHECK ALL RISK FACTORS THAT APPLY. IF ONE OR MORE ITEMS ARE CHECKED, CONSIDER THE PATIENT AT RISK AND INTIATE THE FALL PREVENTION PROTOCOL.

☐ AGE 75 OR MORE
☐ HISTORY OF FALLS
☐ IMPAIRED PHYSICAL STATUS: MOBILITY, DIZZINESS, WEAKNESS, ORTHOSTATIC BLOOD PRESSURE CHANGES

☐ IMPAIRED MENTAL STATUS; CONFUSED
☐ FREQUENT TOILETING: RELATED TO MEDICATIONS/DISEASE
☐ NONE OF THE ABOVE RISK FACTORS PRESENT

ASSESSMENT/**OTHER SIGNIFICANT FINDINGS**

SIGNIFICANT OTHER

CHECK ALL THAT APPLY:

☐ SIGNIFICANT OTHER WILL BE INVOLVED IN THE ONGOING TREATMENT PLAN. STATE RELATIONSHIP: _____
☐ SIGNIFICANT OTHER CONTRIBUTED TO THIS ASSESSMENT.
☐ PATIENT HAS NO SIGNIFICANT OTHER OR SIGNIFICANT OTHER UNKNOWN.

ADDITIONAL COMMENTS:

RN SIGNATURE AND TITLE: _____ DATE: _____

PRINT NAME: _____

USE PEN ONLY WHEN COMPLETING THIS FORM. DATE AND INITIAL ALL ENTRIES.
The initial plan of care, including the selection of Standard(s) of Care and Protocols, is based upon review of the information contained in the Nursing Admission Assessment.

STANDARD(S) OF CARE AND PROTOCOLS

Date	Init	(Insert name of applicable standard/protocol)	DC Date	Init	(Insert name of applicable standard/protocol)	DC Date	Init

DISCHARGE PLANNING

Date	Init	Discharge Needs	Comments (date and initial)
		Unable to assess on admission (explain).	
		Discharge to home. No assistance required.	
		Discharge to home with assistance (explain).	
		Discharge to other facility (explain).	
		Other (explain).	

REFERRALS

Date	Init	Department notified (insert name)
		Social Service:
		Nurse Specialist:
		Home Care:
		Dietary:
		Pastoral Care:
		Other (specify):

SIGNIFICANT OTHER

NAME AND RELATIONSHIP:

PATIENT SPECIFIC PROBLEMS

(LIST NURSING DIAGNOSIS/PATIENT CARE PROBLEMS NOT INCLUDED IN THE STANDARD(S) OF CARE AND PROTOCOLS LISTED ABOVE.)

Date	Init	#	Nursing Diagnosis (Problem)	Desired Outcome	Nursing Interventions	Resolved Date	Init

NURSE'S INITIALS, SIGNATURE & TITLE

CHAPTER 13

THE ATTENDING STAFF: SENIOR PHYSICIANS

A hospital's attending staff comprises those physicians who may admit their patients to that hospital for care. For the duration of the hospitalization, the patient's care is directed by the attending physician. The attending staff includes physicians of all the specialties and subspecialties. While the house staff (interns, residents, and fellows) come and go as they complete their years of training, the attending staff remains more constant.

In order to join the attending staff of a hospital, a doctor has to apply for admitting privileges: the authority to admit patients to that hospital and to supervise the care of the patient during the hospitalization. Surgeons with privileges are allowed to perform surgery in the hospital's operating rooms.

In general, hospitals carefully restrict how many physicians in each specialty are granted admitting privileges. The number is determined by how many physicians it takes to keep the hospital beds full, without creating such a demand for beds that it is difficult to admit patients in a timely fashion. The more renowned the hospital, the more difficult it is to be granted admitting privileges.

FULL-TIME AND VOLUNTARY STAFF

In teaching hospitals (and some community hospitals as well) the attending staff is usually divided further into the full-time staff and the voluntary staff.

FULL-TIME STAFF

Full-time staff are doctors who work for the hospital. They may have a variety of financial arrangements, but in the final analysis, the hospital acts as their employer.

Attending physicians who are on the full-time staff at a medical school-affiliated hospital also have teaching positions that mirror those of any university. They begin their careers as instructors. As they are promoted, titles are assistant professor, associate professor, full professor, and finally, after retirement, emeritus professor. Every promotion brings increased prestige, responsibilities, and income.

Teaching responsibilities may include both classroom teaching (during the first two years of medical school) and bedside teaching. As noted in the next chapter, during the first two years of medical school, most learning takes place in classrooms. Students are taught basic sciences (anatomy, biochemistry, histology, microbiology, pharmacology, physiology) and rarely spend time with patients. Clinical, or bedside, teaching involves supervising medical students and house officers as they care for patients in the hospital or outpatient setting.

Frequently, the full-time staff is further broken down into clinical and research staff. While the distinction between the two groups is often blurred, research faculty generally spend most of their time in the laboratory, while clinical faculty take care of patients.

Both full-time and voluntary attendings in each specialty are grouped into departments. For example, all the internists in the hospital are members of the department of internal medicine, which is responsible for the administration of the medical service. The department chair (a full professor) is powerful and decides who gets admitting privileges, who is promoted, what the salary levels are, and who does the teaching.

Each subspecialty in the department of internal medicine (e.g., cardiology, gastroenterology, hematology, endocrinology) is organized along the same lines into a division. The chair of the division of cardiology has the same general responsibilities as the chair of medicine, but in a more localized fiefdom. Division chairs report to and are guided by the department chair.

VOLUNTARY STAFF

The voluntary (private practitioner) staff are physicians who have opened their own medical practice and are financially responsible for themselves. In many ways, they are small-business owners. They can admit their patients to the hospital, direct their care, and participate in medical research and teaching, but overall, they are self-employed professionals.

Community hospitals may have a small full-time staff, but most of their physicians are voluntary. Some hospitals, such as the Mayo Clinic, have only full-time physicians and no outside physician can admit a patient. Outside physicians may, however, refer patients to the clinic, in which case a Mayo Clinic attending physician will be assigned to the patient for the duration of the stay.

Until the 1960s, most attending physicians in this country were general practitioners, doctors who could do a little bit of everything. This required four years of medical school followed by a "rotating internship"—two- to three-month blocks of time on each of the five major teaching services in the hospital (internal medicine, surgery, pediatrics, psychiatry, and obstetrics/gynecology). Physicians could then open an office and they were all set to begin their practice. But as medicine became increasingly complex, medical students were urged to pursue additional training, and organized medicine moved into the age of the internist and general surgeon as the primary caregivers. More recently, with ever more knowledge needed to handle many problems, many medical students opt to become subspecialists.

SPECIALISTS

INTERNISTS

To become an internist and practice general internal medicine requires three years of training after medical school, in an accredited hospital training program. This includes one year of internship and two subsequent years of residency, all on an internal medicine service in a hospital. To then become a medical subspecialist requires several more years of training in an accredited hospital program that is exclusively dedicated to that subspecialty. For example, it takes three additional years of training in cardiology, after three years of internal medicine, to be certified as a cardiologist. Thus, the cardiologist's entire post–high school education—including four years of college, four years of medical school, three years of internship and residency, and three further years of fellowship training in cardiology—totals fourteen years. The same rigorous training is required by other medical subspecialties, which include cardiology, endocrinology, gastroenterology, hematology, nephrology, neurology, oncology, and pulmonology.

After physicians complete each stage of training, they are allowed to take the nationally administered examinations. Each subspecialty has a board of governors who are elected for varying terms. The governors select a board of medical examiners who are responsible for the content and administration of the national board examinations. Thus, a physician who passes the exam is "board certified." Physicians can take the exam in more than one area; for example, some hematologists are also board certified in immunology.

The initials that appear after a doctor's name signify his or her training and any board certification. For example, John Smith, MD, FACP, FACC, stands for John Smith, Medical Doctor, Fellow of the American College of Physicians and Fellow of the American College of Cardiology. This means that Dr. Smith has passed the examinations required to be certified as an internist and as a cardiologist and is therefore accepted into the medical societies that govern these groups of physicians. Not all physicians and surgeons display their initials even when board certified. So ask!

One small disclaimer is needed, however. Board certification is no guarantee of superior quality, and a number of excellent doctors have never bothered to become board certified.

**BECOMING A
CARDIOLOGIST**

College 4 years
Medical School 4 years
Internship 1 year
Residency 2 years
Fellowship 3 years
Total: 14 years after
high school

**SURGICAL SPECIALTIES
WITH FULL GENERAL
SURGERY TRAINING**

General surgery
Vascular surgery
Cardiothoracic surgery
Plastic and reconstructive
surgery
Pediatric surgery
Trauma and burn surgery
(specialty fellowships exist,
but independent boards are
not yet formed)

SURGEONS

Surgical specialty training is similar to that of the medical specialties. The surgical equivalent of the internist is the general surgeon. In reality, however, in this day and age, general surgeons in large metropolitan areas tend to be specialists, too, mainly operating on the abdomen and the breast. Many surgical subspecialties have taken over the care of certain other types of surgical procedures. Until the 1960s, a general surgeon could be expected to take out a lung tumor, perform a hysterectomy, or repair a leaking artery. Today, vascular surgeons operate on the major arteries, head-and-neck surgeons take care of tumors of that region, and so on for most of the other areas of the body. What has remained constant is that many of the surgical subspecialties still require that a surgeon complete general surgical training before entering specialty training. Some of the surgical subspecialties, however, require only the first one-to-three years instead of the full five years.

The surgical specialties all have their own national board with examinations for board certification. Surgical training is slightly longer than that for the internal medicine specialties. For example, while general surgery training is five years, cardiothoracic surgery (qualifying to operate on the heart and lungs) requires training for another two years for a total of seven years following medical school.

Sub-subspecialties exist in surgery as well. Cardiac surgeons may do an additional year of training in pediatric cardiac surgery. Plastic and reconstructive surgeons may, after five to seven years of training, do additional fellowships in hand surgery, microvascular surgery, or craniofacial surgery.

PSYCHIATRISTS

Training to become a psychiatrist begins with a one-year internship in internal medicine or a one-year rotating internship (three-month stints in medicine, surgery, obstetrics, and pediatrics). The internship is followed by three years of hospital training in general psychiatry. Subspecialty training such as psychoanalysis may take up to seven more years.

OBSTETRICS/GYNECOLOGY

Four years of training after medical school are required to become an obstetrician/gynecologist. The basic training is somewhat longer than other specialties because it requires expertise in both the delivery and operating rooms. Subspecialty training is less common than in other fields, but does exist; two such subspecialties are high-risk obstetrics and infertility.

SURGICAL SPECIALTIES THAT DO NOT REQUIRE FIVE YEARS OF GENERAL SURGERY TRAINING

Urology
Orthopedics
Otolaryngology (ENT)
Neurosurgery
Plastic and reconstructive surgery

PEDIATRICS

Pediatricians are internists for children. Their training is the same as that for internists in length, complexity, and ultimate subspecialization. Pediatricians complete a general pediatric residency, then enter pediatric subspecialty training, and require no training in adult medicine. In contrast, pediatric surgeons require the full five years of training in adult general surgery, and then receive an additional two years of training in pediatric surgery.

CHAPTER 14

YOUR HOSPITAL TEAM

The surgeon, internist, or other specialist who is in charge of your surgery or treatment is not the only person who follows your daily progress. The hospital assigns each patient an entire team of caregivers who are familiar with that patient's needs and who provide or monitor his or her care. The various people who waft in and out of your room in their white coats, either alone or as a group during morning rounds, are members of your team. And each team is part of a "service": a group of doctors, nurses, therapists, administrators, secretaries, and other personnel who deal with one specific aspect of medical care.

Major services or departments include internal medicine, surgery, pediatrics, psychiatry, and obstetrics/gynecology. Specialty services are divisions of the departments and include such subspecialties as urology, ophthalmology, ENT (ear, nose, and throat), orthopedics, neurology, plastic surgery, and dermatology.

Teams vary according to their service. For example, medical, pediatric, and psychiatric service teams usually include the head nurse on the floor, one or more medical students, interns, residents, and a teaching attending physician. On surgical, obstetrics, and gynecology services, the team is composed of the chief resident, interns, residents, medical students, nurses, and, frequently, physician's assistants.

Following is a description of the physicians on your team.

THE HOUSE STAFF: INTERNS, RESIDENTS, AND FELLOWS

Every patient admitted to the hospital is assigned to one intern and generally one resident. Both take a history and conduct a physical examination upon the patient's arrival, and remain responsible for the patient's care for the duration of the hospitalization. They write notes in the patient's chart, order tests, draw blood, and handle other day-to-day aspects of the patient's care, such as collecting test results and monitoring bowel problems. Interns, residents, and fellows are collectively known as the house staff, or house officers.

The house-staff hierarchy has not changed in fifty years. Some years ago, there was a move to eliminate the word *intern* and replace it with *first-year resident* for medicine and *PGY1* (postgraduate year one) for surgery. It soon became obvious that a rose by any other name remains a rose, and we returned to the classical nomenclature.

Following is a brief description of the duties and training of the various members of a house-staff team.

> **"THE TEAM"**
>
> **Attending physician**
> **Fellow**
> **Chief resident**
> **Senior resident**
> **Resident**
> **Intern**
> **Physician's assistant**
> **Nurse**
> **Medical student**
> **Therapists (occupational, physical, or respiratory)**

MEDICAL STUDENTS

Third- and fourth-year medical students are an integral part of hospital teams. They have completed most of their book learning and are aching to participate in actual patient care. Third-year medical students are frequently assigned to examine and interview patients with interesting and unusual problems. Patients frequently see this as an intrusion and feel that they are being used as "guinea pigs." While it is true that the students are learning from every case they see, they frequently add crucial medical knowledge, because in an attempt to learn and shine, they often rush to the medical library after seeing patients. They read all of the latest articles pertaining to certain problems and are eager to share their new knowledge with the rest of the team.

INTERNS

An intern is a newly minted physician who has just graduated from an accredited medical school; that is, one that has met standards set by the American Association of Medical Colleges. The AAMC requires medical schools to have a certain number of faculty members; offer coverage of basic medical material; provide sufficient exposure to patients; and maintain adequate lab facilities. An intern has had two years of classroom training in the basic sciences and two further years of clinical practice taking care of patients on the various hospital services. Many are terrified in July, when they begin their internship, and cocky in June, when they are about to become residents. They are responsible for knowing everything about the patients to whom they are assigned, and do all the "scut" work involved in patient care. This pejorative hospital term refers to the busy tasks of ordering tests, checking lab data, drawing blood, starting IVs, and writing copious notes in the patient's chart.

There is a curious misconception in our country that these young doctors should be avoided because they are "just learning" and "are practicing on patients." Learning? Yes. Practicing? Never to the detriment of the patient and always under supervision. The bottom line is that the house staff is a major safety factor for the patients. First of all, there is a house officer in the hospital who is responsible for each patient twenty-four hours a day. Attending physicians can only spend a portion of every day in the hospital. The rest of the time, they are either taking care of people in their private offices or are off duty (frequently reachable by beeper, but not physically present in the hospital). If you need emergency care when your attending physician is unavailable, it is reassuring to have a house officer available immediately who knows your situation.

Additionally, these young physicians are fresh out of medical school and have been imbued with the latest knowledge about a wide variety of diseases. There is an unwritten, unspoken competition between house staff and attending physicians that ultimately benefits the patient. In an effort to impress or one-up the senior physician, the younger doctors try to find a new diagnosis that has not been considered or a new treatment that they have just learned about. There's a cliché that "two heads are better than one"; certainly, when you are ill, the more people thinking about your problem, the better. So when a fresh-faced young doctor comes over, don't be chagrined, but recognize the attention as part of the greatness of the university teaching hospital.

In the past, university hospitals discouraged house officers from being married. An intern was practically expected to live in the hospital, and was grudgingly allowed only a few hours off every third day. The hours are not as brutal now, but the responsibility of being in charge of a patient's life remains awesome and motivating.

RESIDENTS

The hallmark of being a resident is the ability to use the "royal *we*."

"Why don't we do an EKG on Mrs. Jones?" translates into: "Intern, do an EKG."

Residents supervise the minute-to-minute work of the interns. Residents are expected to read the latest medical information about their current cases, impart this knowledge to the interns (and sometimes to the senior physicians as well), and help with any complicated procedures, such as spinal taps.

The duration of residency training differs depending on the specialty. For example, an internist spends one year as an intern and two subsequent years as a resident; a general surgeon spends one year as an intern and four years as a resident.

FELLOWS

After completing an internship and a residency, physicians may choose to further subspecialize. An internist may decide to become a cardiologist; a general surgeon may opt to learn plastic surgery. Doctors who are in training in these subspecialties may still be called residents but are often known as fellows, and the amount of time they spend in training varies according to the regulations of each subspecialty's governing body. Fellowships are difficult to obtain, especially in the more popular fields such as dermatology, cardiac surgery, and ophthalmology.

ATTENDING PHYSICIANS

An attending physician is a doctor who has graduated from medical school, completed at least an internship, and been granted admitting privileges at a hospital.

It is legal for people to get a medical license and then practice any specialty they please, without necessarily obtaining extra training. In reality, this is rarely done because of the changing nature of internships, and the regulatory brake applied by credentialing and quality-assurance committees.

THE CHANGING NATURE OF INTERNSHIPS

Internships today are quite different in character from the "rotating internships" that prevailed until the 1970s. During rotating internships, physicians spent two- to three-month blocks of time on a variety of hospital services. They performed minor operations, delivered babies, treated heart attacks, and occasionally even rendered psychiatric care. Not only did these internships constitute the standard of care and training for that time; they were also adequate to transmit the requisite fund of knowledge for that era. The internships were genuinely intended to teach, not to be "medical smorgasbords" that let physicians sample different aspects of medical care.

Today, however, with the explosion of medical knowledge and the prevalence of subspecialties, internships no longer suffice as stand-alone training programs. Medicine has become so complicated that it is just impossible to learn enough after one year to deliver any sort of safe, quality medicine. Rotating internships still exist, but only as a prerequisite for *subsequent* training in such specialties as psychiatry, obstetrics and gynecology, and ophthalmology. The old-time GP is a vanishing breed. Family practitioners may resemble GPs, but they are really specialists themselves. They have to undergo a three-year training program in family practice, including all areas of medicine (surgery, pediatrics, obstetrics and gynecology, and so forth) and periodic reexamination in order to achieve and maintain the certification.

QUALITY-ASSURANCE AND CREDENTIALING COMMITTEES

Quality-assurance committees review hospital procedures to make sure they are being done safely. For example, if an intern performs a spinal tap and the patient has a complication, the quality-assurance committee reviews the event and may establish a rule that no interns should perform the procedure without supervision until they have performed five under supervision. Or if a patient has died following an angioplasty, the quality-assurance committee investigates and may find that between the angioplasty lab and the intensive care unit, the patient was alone with a transport worker. The committee may direct that all patients who have had angioplasties must be transported by catheterization lab physicians.

The quality-assurance committee is made up of physicians in a specialty such as internal medicine, as well as representatives from the subspecialties. If they find that a certain physician is responsible for many problems, they have the power to suggest removal of his or her privileges by the department chairman. The committee's deliberations may be subpoenaed during discovery (a legal procedure) in a malpractice case. If the committee finds that a physician has made a mistake, it is hard to defend the case.

Credentialing Committees are generally part of the medical board and may use information from Quality Assurance Committees for appointments and reappointments.

OTHER TEAM MEMBERS

At some point during your hospital admission, you may be visited by such other members of your team as therapists, dieticians, social workers, and/or clergy. Others, such as pharmacists, "visit" you without entering your room by checking your doctor's orders and reading your hospital chart.

THERAPISTS

Following surgery and during many medical admissions, a therapist can provide invaluable assistance with your recovery. There are three main categories of therapists: respiratory, occupational, and physical.

Respiratory therapists deal with the function of your lungs. They help patients who are recuperating from surgery or who are in prolonged bed rest to keep their lungs in working order (full of air and free of fluid). Lungs are filled with air sacs called alveoli. Problems occur if the alveoli fill with fluid or collapse entirely. This may occur with infection or mainly with failure to take deep breaths because of pain after surgery. Patients whose lung function is compromised are susceptible to pneumonia and may not oxygenate their red blood cells adequately. Respiratory therapists help by instructing patients in coughing and deep breathing by strongly tapping or massaging the patient's chest and back to help keep the alveoli open. Oxygen gets into the lungs and then into the blood.

Physical therapists help patients to regain use of their limbs and to ambulate (walk) following prolonged illness or surgery. Physical therapists may use passive motion, show patients how to do exercises for improving the mobility and activity of joints, or instruct them on how to use canes, crutches, and walkers. They also teach people who are bedridden how to do movements that maintain the full range of motion, so that their joints don't become too stiff.

Occupational therapists often work closely with surgeons in caring for patients with hand injuries or paralysis secondary to strokes. This care requires the use of special splints to hold the hand in a certain position, to encourage it to open up more, or to gently rehabilitate a healing tendon. Occupational therapists' ability to fabricate these custom splints out of a plasticlike material has also made occupational therapists important members of teams that care for burn patients.

PHARMACISTS

One of the most important professionals involved in your care is someone you will absolutely never see and never get a bill from. The hospital pharmacist makes sure that patients receive the medications ordered by their physicians. The pharmacist checks that you have no abnormal drug interactions, reviews your history of allergies to make sure you can receive the ordered drugs without a reaction, and mixes intravenous fluids and special orders.

Yet no matter how many thousands of times pharmacists, nurses, and others check orders and medications, mistakes can occasionally occur. *Always check everything that goes into your mouth.* If you are not sure, ask the nurse or one of your doctors before swallowing any pill.

CHAPTER 15

DOCTORS BEHIND THE SCENES

N ot long after you leave the hospital, your mailbox will fill with medical bills. You certainly expect bills from your primary physician and any specialists consulted on your diagnosis or care—but you may be surprised to find bills from physicians you don't know. Although these bills may seem to surface out of nowhere, hospitals have a number of "behind-the-scenes" physicians who play crucial, though little-known, roles in determining diagnosis and directing treatment. In the past, most of these charges were included in a single hospital bill, but government regulations now mandate a separate interpretation fee and, therefore, a separate bill.

Behind-the-scenes doctors from whom you might receive a separate bill may include physiatrists, emergency room attending physicians, intensivists, radiologists, and pathologists.

PHYSIATRISTS

Physiatrists are physicians who specialize in rehabilitation of the body (not to be confused with psychiatrists, whose arena is the mind). Physiatrists design and direct rehabilitation programs for patients with such problems as strokes and fractures; supervise postoperative mobilization;

and oversee the treatment provided by occupational and physical therapists.

EMERGENCY ROOM ATTENDING PHYSICIANS

Emergency room attending physicians are part of a recent formed specialty of emergency medicine. Interestingly, they are a throwback to the old idea of the general practitioner, trained in a bit of everything. They deal with trauma, childbirth, heart attacks, and more—all in one day. While this makes for an exciting life, it is at the expense of long-term relationships with patients.

INTENSIVISTS

Intensivists are specialists in critical care medicine, and are typically the full-time physician staff of intensive care units. If you have been a patient in an intensive care unit, you were probably seen by hordes of physicians whose names and faces have blurred, and you may not remember the intensivist in particular. But it was this physician who made the minute-to-minute, life-and-death decisions that had to be made on the spot, and who consulted with your attending physician on the best approach to your care.

RADIOLOGISTS

Radiologists are physicians who specialize in the performance and reading of X rays. At one time, radiologists rarely interacted with patients, but spent most of their time in front of a lighted view box where they read and interpreted X rays, then forwarded their findings to the primary physician. Many radiologists continue to work that way, but some have expanded their role, becoming "interventional radiologists" who actively participate in treatment as well as diagnosis.

Consider, for example, the case of a patient who has smoked heavily for a long time and now complains of severe leg pains whenever he walks. An X ray reveals that he has blockages in the arteries that supply blood to his legs. A condition called arteriosclerosis has caused a narrowing in the diameter of the arteries, reducing the flow of blood to the tissues of his leg and causing pain while walking, a condition called intermittent claudication.

In the past, the only treatments were medical therapy or major surgery. A vascular surgeon would have to bypass the blocked section of artery with a section of artificial tubing and/or a vein graft. But today, a radiologist can perform an angioplasty to correct the patient's condition without the need for major surgery. In this procedure, which is done in a radiology suite under sterile conditions, an interventional radiologist, or "angiographer," inserts a small catheter into an artery, and under radiographic guidance, places the end of the catheter at the site of the blockage. The end of the catheter has a balloon that the radiologist inflates at the site of the blockage, squashing the obstruction, thus opening the artery and improving blood flow and relieving pain.

Interventional radiologists can aid physicians and surgeons in many other ways as well. They perform biopsies of deep tumors or pass needles to drain fluid collections and infections. Where once radiologists could only visualize deep into the body, now they are capable of intervening deep into the body without the need for an extensive surgical procedure.

PATHOLOGISTS

These medical doctors specialize in analyzing and studying human tissues, cells, and fluids. The pathology subspecialties most likely to be pertinent to your care are surgical and clinical pathology.

A surgical pathologist examines tissue (skin, muscle, bone, intestine, etc.) and cells through a microscope in order to diagnose disease. A biopsy is the surgical removal of tissue for analysis by a pathologist. The most thorough analysis of tissue may take several days, and requires the tissue specimen to be prepared and processed in a prescribed, sophisticated manner called a "permanent section."

However, there are times when a surgeon cannot wait several days and needs the analysis right away. For example, if a patient is in the operating room and a surgeon has just removed some tissue, the remainder of the operation may hinge on whether the pathologist identifies the tissue as malignant.

In these critical situations—which may include procedures for such problems as breast or skin cancer, head or neck tumors, or a growth on an ovary—the pathologists prepare the tissue as a "frozen section." This technique is not as accurate as permanent sections, but it takes minutes instead of days. Nevertheless, it is much more difficult for the pathologist to interpret the tissue because its appearance under the microscope is not as detailed or clear as that of a permanent section. It is, however, an expected risk of frozen sections that the percentage of inaccuracies is higher than with permanent sections. Pathologists and surgeons will not proceed with more extensive procedures on the basis of frozen sections if there is any doubt as to the diagnosis, a practice that reduces but does not completely eliminate the chance of error.

Clinical pathologists run the laboratories where the blood tests are processed. Their fees are included with the charges for your laboratory tests, so they do not send a separate bill. Some of the most common blood tests performed pertain to the blood count, blood chemistries, sugar levels, liver and kidney functioning, cholesterol and lipids, and blood clotting. (See the Glossary of Procedures.)

Another pathology specialty that has gotten much attention is forensic pathology, the performance of autopsies that may help reveal the cause(s), nature, and time of death. Autopsies generally reveal which organs and tissues are involved with disease, whether related to the cause of death or not. The tissues and blood can also be analyzed for the presence of poisons, drugs, or medications. The media often portray these pathologists aiding the police in the investigation of crimes. One hopes they will have no role in your hospitalization!

The doctors behind the scenes play a significant role in the delivery of your care while in the hospital. Your well-being is their concern, and they are as important as your private physician to the efficient and effective resolution of your medical problems.

CHAPTER 16

ANESTHESIA AND PAIN MANAGEMENT

For centuries, surgical procedures were done with no anesthesia other than a swig of brandy or a numbing of the area with ice, and no distraction other than biting on a silver bullet. Surgery was usually performed only when death was the only other alternative, and often people passed out from the pain.

About a century ago, however, physicians in an amphitheater at the Massachusetts General Hospital in Boston ushered in a new era of medicine when they witnessed the first use of ether as an anesthetic; to this day, the amphitheater is known as the Ether Dome.

Ether and other forms of anesthesia dramatically improved surgical outcomes, made new and lengthier surgical procedures possible, and eventually expanded surgery to include elective, rather than only emergency, surgery.

Today, there are many types of anesthetic agents and sedatives that reduce pain, sedate or relax you, induce a state of amnesia regarding the surgery if you remain conscious, or render you totally unconscious in the case of general anesthesia.

MEETING YOUR ANESTHESIOLOGIST

Your anesthetist (the person responsible for your anesthesia) may be a physician (anesthesiologist) or a registered nurse (a CRNA, or Certified Registered Nurse Anesthetist). In most hospitals, a small group of anesthesiologists tend to work with a specific surgical service, thereby creating a group of anesthesia subspecialists. For example, a group of anesthesiologists might work almost exclusively with orthopedic surgeons. Other examples of subspecializations are cardiac, obstetrical, pediatric, intensive care unit, and pain management anesthesiologists. Such specialization works to patients' advantage, since smooth coordination between the surgeon and the anesthesiologist makes every part of the operation more efficient, safe, and comfortable for the patient.

Nurse anesthetists in hospitals work under an anesthesiologist's supervision. In many free-standing surgi-centers and offices, nurse anesthetists may work independently. For many types of anesthesia, such as intravenous sedation (also called local-standby or MAC, monitored anesthesia care), they perform as well as anesthesiologists. For more complicated procedures, such as specialized blocks or cardiac anesthesia, the presence of an anesthesiologist is mandatory but a CRNA often assists.

In many instances, an anesthesiologist is assigned to a case on the afternoon or evening before surgery, according to who is scheduled to be on duty at the time of surgery. However, you may be surprised to learn that you and your surgeon may not be required to accept the "luck of the draw." Some hospitals permit surgeons to request a specific anesthesiologist. Patients should always have the right to choose their own anesthesiologist, but unless they or someone they know have had a particular anesthesiologist previously, they are not usually informed consumers. Therefore, the best approach is to ask the surgeon to recommend an experienced, board certified anesthesiologist with whom the surgeon has worked on similar cases. In fact, surgeons have been known to hold up the start of surgery when unhappy with the anesthesia coverage. A surgeon is, after all, the "captain of the ship" and ultimately responsible for all aspects of an operation.

When and where you will first meet the anesthesiologist varies not only by institution but also according to the type of procedure for which you are scheduled.

For *ambulatory, same-day procedures*, for which you are admitted to the hospital the day of surgery and discharged the same day or within twenty-three hours of admission, you may meet with an attending anesthesiologist when you have your preadmission testing performed. This physician will not necessarily be the anesthesiologist who will be present at your operation; the purpose of this meeting is to assess your anesthesia risk and to determine if any additional testing (e.g., arterial blood gases or specialized medical consultation by a cardiologist) may be necessary.

For *traditional admission*, for which you are admitted on the day prior to surgery, you usually meet the anesthesiologist the evening before surgery. You and your surgeon already should have had some discussion regarding the choices of anesthetic techniques. The meeting with the anesthesiologist is your opportunity to discuss your options and preferences and the risks and advantages of various anesthetic techniques. Do not hesitate to ask questions and express concerns. Although the anesthesiologist will have limited time to describe the full range of anesthetic techniques, you should certainly receive answers to the following questions:

- What are my anesthesia options?
- Which type of anesthesia do you recommend? Why?
- What are my risks?
- How will I feel after the anesthesia?
- What do I have to do to prepare for anesthesia?
- How will I be monitored? Do you use a pulse oximeter and a CO_2 expiratory gas monitor?

PRE-ANESTHESIA TESTING

The laboratory tests required by anesthesiologists are the same as those ordered by your surgeon. The anesthesiologist will use your EKG and chest X ray to assess the functioning of your heart and lungs. Your normal blood work will also help indicate whether you are healthy enough to undergo surgery and are not at increased risk for any specific anesthetic technique.

Since you generally meet with an anesthesiologist on the day that your preoperative testing is performed, the anesthesiologist will not

---

IMPORTANT PRECAUTIONS BEFORE ANESTHESIA

If you have ever had any allergies or other problems with any anesthesia or medications, be sure to tell both your surgeon and anesthesiologist.

Tell the anesthesiologist which medications, vitamins, or other supplements you are taking.

Specify if you have any temporary caps, removable bridges, loose teeth, or orthodontic appliances so that the anesthesiologist will make sure they are not swallowed or damaged.

Give your dentures to a family member or a nurse on the floor or the admitting area before proceeding to the holding area or the operating room.

Make sure you have not had anything to eat or drink. You don't want anything in your stomach that can be aspirated into your lungs.

---

have these results available to review until the next day or later. If the anesthesiologist finds an abnormal value or something else of concern, you may need additional testing or medical clearance. *Don't be alarmed* if you get a phone call to this effect. In most cases, this does not indicate any new or serious illness, nor does it even delay or cancel the procedure. The most common reasons for repeat of a test are that the lab made an error or lost the specimen.

THE ANESTHESIA REPERTOIRE

General anesthesia. Also called being "put to sleep," this is the most complete and deepest form of anesthesia. It consists of three components: total loss of consciousness with resultant amnesia of the operative procedure; complete loss of voluntary movement; and total analgesia (freedom from pain). The anesthesiologist assumes full monitoring and control of the patient's functioning. It is the anesthesiologist's role to administer anesthesia properly, to keep careful watch during surgery, and to bring the patient out of anesthesia safely.

The main risk of general anesthesia is that patients can lose not only the ability to breathe for themselves, but also involuntary protective reflexes. One such reflex normally prevents solids and liquids from going through the larynx and into the lungs—a common experience most people refer to as having something "go down the wrong pipe." The loss of the reflex during general anesthesia is important, since its failure to function can put a person at risk of aspirating (breathing in) stomach contents that may be vomited. This can lead to "aspiration pneumonia," a serious condition. Therefore, the anesthesiologist usually places an "endotracheal tube" down your throat and through your trachea in order to guarantee complete control of your breathing and to protect your lungs from aspiration. The tube guarantees the delivery of oxygen and anesthetic gases to the proper location, your lungs, and helps seal the entrance to your lungs from any stomach fluids that might enter and cause damage. To guide the placement of the tube through the vocal cords into the trachea, the anesthesiologist uses a *laryngoscope*, an instrument that aids in proper exposure, alignment, and lighting.

The endotracheal tube provides valuable protection, but it irritates the lining of the trachea. That's why so many patients complain of a sore throat after general anesthesia. Another potential problem is that the pressure of the laryngoscope against the lower jaw can place a patient's dental work at risk.

If a person is having a short procedure (less than one hour) and does not need to be moved during the operation, the anesthetist sometimes does not insert an endotracheal tube but controls respiration with a rubber face mask that resembles the mask with which an airline flight attendant demonstrates safety. The risk of face mask anesthesia is that the trachea is not protected from aspiration, and the airway is dependent on the continued proper placement of the face mask by the anesthesiologist. More recently developed endotracheal tubes have a "minimask" at the end of the endotracheal tube in an attempt to combine the benefits of both of the other tubes with fewer of the risks.

The depth of general anesthesia is maintained through either gases that people breathe in (inspired gases) or intravenous agents (medications). While careful monitoring of these substances is important throughout surgery, the periods of greatest risk are at the beginning, for the several minutes when the patient is being induced or put to sleep, and at the end, when the patient is being awakened. As one medical school professor put it, putting a patient to sleep is like flying a plane; the most difficult parts are the take-off and landing. It is important to remember, however, that statistically, flying in a commercial plane is safer than crossing the street in a big city. The same goes for anesthesia. The incidence of serious complications is very, very rare.

Regional anesthesia. This method renders the appropriate area free from pain by delivering an anesthetic agent directly to the individual nerve or nerve bundle that supplies that area; this technique is most frequently employed for orthopedic and obstetrical procedures. For example, patients who are undergoing a total knee replacement or having a cesarean section are candidates for an *epidural* anesthesia, one type of regional anesthesia. Other common forms of regional anesthesia are spinal, axillary block, scalene block, digital, wrist, and ankle block. By placing a needle in the epidural space just outside the spinal cord, the anesthesiologist can numb the patient from the waist down. Regional anesthesia can numb an area from one to six hours, depending on the anesthetic agent and methods employed. In some instances, an epidural catheter is left in place. For longer procedures, more anesthetic agent can be reintroduced to extend the duration of the anesthesia. In addition, pain medication can be delivered through the epidural catheter for more effective analgesia (pain relief).

Local anesthesia. The direct injection of local anesthesia into a particular site is the simplest form of anesthesia. Every physician, physician's assistant, and dentist who performs a procedure administers local anesthesia. Although many patients refer to local anesthesia as "novocaine," novocaine is rarely used today because of a high incidence of allergic reactions. More common is the local anesthetic agent lidocaine.

Standby anesthesia. This is the use of various intravenous anesthetic agents to complement local and regional anesthesia, making the patient more relaxed and producing analgesia and amnesia. This combination of anesthetic techniques is also referred to as MAC (monitored anesthesia care). A combination of anesthetic agents, pain relievers, and sedatives is delivered through a running intravenous line both prior to the injection of the local/regional anesthesia and during the procedure. The medications help to relax the patient and to provide additional pain relief and amnesia during the procedure.

THE DIFFERENCES AMONG LOCAL, TOPICAL, AND REGIONAL ANESTHESIA

Local anesthesia is the superficial injection of an anesthetic agent directly into the area that needs to be anesthetized. It is administered into the skin by needle.

Topical anesthesia is the application of an anesthetic agent onto mucosal (wet) surfaces such as gum or cornea by rubbing into the area or giving drops. An anesthesetic agent works only on those areas it directly touches. The dose during any one time period is limited, due to toxicity.

Regional, or block anesthesia is the injection of an anesthetic agent in order to block, or anesthetize, a main or central nerve that connects to the peripheral sensory nerve endings in a particular part of the body, thus rendering that part of the body numb. It permits anesthetization of much larger areas of the body than does local anesthesia, thus reducing the risk of overdose. This method requires a higher level of skill and involves greater risks, since the needle goes deeper into the body than with local anesthesia.

DECIDING ABOUT ANESTHESIA

The rule of thumb for choosing anesthesia is that one should choose the safest and simplest anesthesia that is suitable for the procedure and for the patient.

No anesthetic technique is right for every person or every procedure. Just as the anesthesiologist has to know the proper agents and techniques for each surgical procedure, patients have to have some sense of their own anxiety and pain threshold. Some people find the concept of any degree of awareness of the sights or sounds associated with a surgical procedure impossible to tolerate; they may be better off either heavily sedated or under general anesthesia. Others do not seem to be troubled by the surgical environment and can be anesthetized more lightly.

In general, *the simpler the anesthesia, the safer it is and the better you feel afterward.* A hip replacement using a regional anesthetic technique is associated with fewer anesthetic complications than one using general anesthesia. Overall, there has been a trend away from using general anesthesia. Discuss the choices with your surgeon and anesthetist, consider your own preferences, and, when possible, opt for local or regional anesthesia for quicker recovery and fewer complications and risks.

PAIN MANAGEMENT

Pain management is a relatively recent subspecialty of anesthesia that now plays a significant role in the care of patients not only during their surgery, but during their convalescence as well. Many anesthesiologists spend all or a lot of their time on pain management. They may help a patient who is in extreme pain after surgery through means such as these:

- Their medications are replaced with more effective ones.
- Special pumps are provided that allow the patient to self-medicate as needed (within safety limits, of course).
- Special lines are placed, such as epidural catheters, that deliver pain medication directly to the space around the nerves of the spinal cord, thereby alleviating the patient's pain with a lower dosage of medication.

Anesthesiologists also assist patients with chronic pain. Many people, especially those who have been injured in accidents, can develop chronic pain syndromes such as reflex sympathetic dystrophy (RSD). Blocking or anesthetizing the area multiple times during a period of one to several weeks or more can often alleviate or eliminate this problem. Unfortunately, many insurance carriers do not realize the importance of pain management and cover these services inadequately or not at all.

CHAPTER 17

THE OPERATING ROOM

Virtually every patient feels anxious upon entering the operating room. Even surgeons are apprehensive when the roles are reversed and it's their turn to lie on the operating table.

Knowing that surgery is necessary doesn't prevent your heart from beating fast, your breath from becoming quick and shallow, and your fingers from drumming nervously as you mutter, "What am I doing here?" These are normal and understandable reactions, and the operating room staff will do their best to calm and reassure you.

BEFORE SURGERY BEGINS

PREPPING

Preoperative instructions from your surgeon and the presurgery history, physical, blood work, X rays, and other tests are only the first part of preparation for surgery. In addition to avoiding food or drink, you may also need "prepping"—certain procedures that must be done as close to the time of your procedure as possible, either in the hospital or at home.

Skin prep. Skin washing and shaving of the operative site is done to minimize the chance of infection. Patients used to be shaved by an orderly or nurse's aide the night before surgery. Today, however, you will be shaved by an orderly in the holding area or by the surgeon in the operating room; shaving immediately before the procedure lessens the chance of bacteria "hiding out" in any microscopic nicks that might occur during the shaving.

Bowel prep. The use of oral laxatives and enemas is to help empty the bowels of those who will undergo certain surgical procedures on their intestines. A patient may be given a self-administered enema or, for a more extensive prep, a nurse or nurse's aide will assist.

Bowel preps are done for several reasons. During the operation, stool is less likely to contaminate the surgical field, and the surgical exposure (what surgeons are able to see) is improved because the surgeons do not have to manipulate and retract loops of bowel that are full of stool. Bowel preps promote healing by reducing the fecal stream that would pass any healing wound in the bowel during the first few postoperative days. And since bowels temporarily stop functioning for a few days after surgery, patients are more comfortable if their bowels are empty.

PREMEDICATION

Going to the operating room is somewhat akin to air travel: They rush you onto the plane and then you wait on the runway forever. You know it's almost time to "pull away from the gate" when a nurse comes in with your premedication, one or more drugs (depending on your procedure and anesthesia) given prior to surgery, usually by injection. Drugs are given for several purposes:

- Sedation is the most reliable and effective way to help you relax and overcome your natural feelings of anxiety.
- Respiratory tract secretions must be dry if you are going to have general anesthesia, so that the airways will stay open without collecting fluid.
- The chance of infection associated with surgery is reduced through antibiotics.

If you are an inpatient, you will be transferred onto a stretcher from your hospital bed and steered to the operating room holding area. If you are an ambulatory patient, you may be taken there by stretcher or wheelchair, or permitted to "ambulate" (walk).

IN THE OPERATING ROOM

Pre-Op

If you came in by stretcher, you are transferred directly onto the operating table. If you walked into the operating room under your own steam, you unceremoniously climb up onto the operating table by yourself. A nurse checks your identification bracelet and chart to make sure that you are who they think you are, that your lab data are correct, and that your informed consent form is in the chart.

Now the anesthesiologist takes over, placing EKG electrodes on your chest or back and a blood-pressure cuff on your arm. A pulse oximeter on your finger measures the oxygen saturation of your blood, the amount of oxygen your red blood cells are carrying compared with the maximum they are capable of carrying. An "O^{2}Sat" in the 90-percent range during surgery is considered good. The anesthesiologist also starts an intravenous line and other lines if necessary.

Since you have no clothes on, the operating room may feel chilly, but the thermostat is usually in the 70s. The room is made warmer for burn patients who can suffer rapid loss of body temperature. The anesthesiologist monitors the patient's temperature during long procedures for adults, and during any procedure for children, who tend to lose body heat more rapidly.

To reduce the chance of infection, the OR staff wear caps, masks, special outfits (scrubs), shoe covers or special shoes, and sterile latex gloves and paper surgical gowns for the surgeons and nurses directly involved with the procedure.

To further "de-germ" the environment, you are washed with an antiseptic solution (usually Betadine, an iodine-based solution) and covered with sterile sheets. Anything that comes in contact with the surgical field is sterilized by steam or gas prior to the procedure.

The lights need to be bright to allow maximum illumination of the operative field. If they bother you, ask if they can be adjusted to make you more comfortable.

The surgeons and nurses want you to be as comfortable as possible and will try to put you at ease with light chitchat and friendly smiles. At the same time, the staff does not have a lot of time for hand-holding. Operating rooms are busy places with only one goal in mind: seeing that your surgical procedure is done safely, efficiently, and successfully under the most ideal circumstances. There's not much time for social amenities. If the staff does not seem to spend as much time answering your questions as you would like, do not fear. They have your welfare in mind and are busy making sure that all goes well for you. Nevertheless, *if you have any discomfort whatsoever, tell the nurses or doctors.* Do not be shy.

THE CAST OF CHARACTERS

At least five people are in the operating room: your surgeon and the assistant surgeon, the anesthesiologist, the scrub nurse, and the circulating nurse. In a nonteaching hospital, the surgeon's assistant may be another attending physician on staff, your internist, or a technician. In a teaching or university hospital, the assistant is usually a resident or medical student, and is known as the first assistant. Except for the simplest of surgical procedures, the surgeon needs an assistant to help expose the operative site, control bleeding, and place and cut sutures. For more complicated procedures, second and even third assistants are sometimes necessary.

Scrub nurses hand the proper instruments and suture material to the surgeons during the procedure. They are called scrub nurses because they scrub their hands and don gowns and gloves just as the surgeons do.

Circulating nurses hand extra items needed during the procedure to the scrub nurse, but do not have to scrub or put on a gown. Circulating nurses make sure that the suction machines, cauterization machines, and other equipment are working properly throughout the operation. They also keep count of every sponge, needle, and instrument to make sure that nothing is left inside you. These nurses are generally on their feet throughout the entire procedure and never stop moving, hence the name *circulating* nurse.

Other people in the operating room may be additional surgical assistants (second assistants), additional anesthesiologists, and other nurses and technicians as required by the complexity of the procedure.

TIME TO BEGIN

If you are having general anesthesia, the chapter up to this point describes just about everything you will remember about the operating room. If you are having a regional or local anesthesia, your experience is somewhat different, and you may later recollect some of what transpired from the beginning of anesthesia to the end of surgery.

You may, for example, remember having the surgical field (that portion of the body exposed during surgery) washed with the antiseptic surgical solution, which may feel very cold. (No, it is not kept in a refrigerator.) The surgical field is draped with sterile cloth or cotton sheets to cover the rest of the nonprepped body and to preserve sterility. The surgeon, assistant surgeon, and scrub nurse scrub and put on their gloves and gowns. Surgery begins.

MEMORY'S VACATION

No matter what type of anesthesia you have received, you may have almost no memory of this time in the operating room. Many of the intravenous sedatives used today produce a limited amnesia. Thus, the anxious patient can be sedated to such an extent that his or her lack of recollection of the time spent in the operating room is almost as complete and profound as that of the patient who received a general anesthesia. Some patients, however, are somewhat more relaxed and do not mind being aware of their surroundings and the sequence of events during surgery. If at any point you want more or less sedation, let the anesthesiologist know.

In no case should a patient be uncomfortable or in pain without this being immediately and completely corrected.

A BUSY CONCLUSION

The period at the end of the surgery is somewhat akin to what it must be like to shut down one of the space shuttles after landing; every member of the operating room staff has a set of tasks to perform before the surgery is considered complete and you can be taken to the recovery room. Some patients find the flurry of activity disorienting, but others simply feel relieved that the operation is over, and reassured by the staff's calm and competent handling of this wrap-up phase.

While you lie quietly, still groggy from local anesthesia or perhaps still asleep or just awakening from general anesthesia, the anesthesiologist detaches you from the lines and monitors. The surgeon or assistant surgeon washes the prep solution off you; applies dressings (bandages), casts, etc., and writes the orders for the nurses in the recovery room to follow. The nurses remove the soiled instruments and perform other post-op tasks.

The operating room staff is also busy with paperwork. The nurses keep an operative record for the patient chart; the anesthesiologist maintains an anesthesia record; a surgeon writes a brief operative note in the chart, then dictates a complete report of the operation through the hospital transcription system.

An assistant brings the stretcher into the room, and everybody helps transfer you from the operating room table onto the stretcher. Your surgery is over, and you're off to the recovery room.

PRE-OPERATIVE CHECKLIST

YES = Present/Done N/A = not ordered/				
NO = Is not present not applicable	YES	NO	N/A	REMARKS
CONSENT				
1. CONSENT DATED, SIGNED, WITNESSED				
2. CONSENT CORRESPONDS TO OR SCHEDULE				
A. PATIENT PREPARATION				
3. LANGUAGE: ENGLISH OTHER				
4. PRE-OPERATIVE TEACHING GIVEN & DOCUMENTED				
5. PRE-OP SHOWER OR BATH GIVEN				
6. ENEMA GIVEN				
7. NPO FROM (TIME)				
8. VALUABLES COLLECTED				
9. JEWELRY, COSMETICS, NAIL POLISH, HAIR ACCESSORIES REMOVED				
10. PROSTHESIS REMOVED (DENTURES, BRIDGES, CONTACT LENSES, WIG, OTHER)				
B. SPECIAL PATIENT CONSIDERATIONS				
11. a) BLIND				
b) DEAF				
c) APHASIC				
d) OTHER				
12. DISORIENTATED				
13. LIMITED MOBILITY				
14. ASSISTIVE DEVICES				
a) HEARING AID				
b) CONTACT LENSES				
c) EYE GLASSES				
d) CAPPED TEETH				
e) OTHER				
15. ALLERGIES				
16. ON ISOLATION PRECAUTIONS				
C. SUPPORTIVE LINES & SUPPLIES				
17. a) FOLEY				
b) PERIPHERAL IV				
c) CVP CENTRAL VENOUS PRESSURE				
d) TPN TOTAL PARENTAL NUTRITION				
e) NG TUBE				
f) SWAN GANZ - ARTERIAL LINE				
g) CHEST TUBE/SUCTION DRAINAGE				
h) TRACTION				
i) SPLINTS				
j) DIALYSIS FLUID				
k) PUMPS (INFUSION)				
l) OTHER				
D. CURRENT VITAL SIGNS				
18. a) T P R BP				
b) WEIGHT KG				
19. VOIDED (ON CALL)				
20. PRE-OPERATIVE MEDICATIONS GIVEN/TIME				
21. PRE-OP ANTIBIOTICS OR STEROIDS GIVEN/TIME				
22. PREP DONE AREA: RT. LT. CENTER				
ADDITIONAL COMMENTS				
SIGNATURE & TITLE				

CHECKED BY UNIT NURSE: _____ DATE_____

CHECKED BY O.R. NURSE: _____ DATE_____

	YES	NO	N/A	REMARKS
CHART ORGANIZATION				
LAB RESULTS:				
1. CBC RESULTS				
2. PROTIME				
3. CHEMISTRY				
4. URINALYSIS				
5. EKG				
6. CHEST X RAY				
7. TYPE AND CROSS				
CHART FORMS:				
8. PHYSICAL EXAM SHEET				
9. CONSENT				
10. FACE SHEET				
11. GRAPHIC SHEET				
12. DOCTOR'S ORDER SHEETS				
13. PATIENT'S MEDICATION SHEET				
14. NURSING NOTES OR CRITICAL CARE FLOW SHEET				
15. CHART FORMS IMPRINTED				
16. PATIENT'S ID PLATE ATTACHED				
17. PATIENT'S HISTORY NUMBER CORRESPONDS WITH FACE SHEET, ID BAND				
18. PATIENT'S OLD CHART				

CHECKED BY: _____ SIGNATURE, TITLE

CHECKED BY O.R. NURSE: _____ DATE _____

O.R. COMMENTS: _____

_____

_____

CHAPTER 18

THE RECOVERY ROOM

Surgery is over. You awaken in a bed with rails like an adult-size crib, in a large, noisy room. You're conscious, yet not fully alert; you may feel disoriented, off-kilter, confused, perhaps, by the commotion around you. Oddly, you may also feel happier than you have ever been in your entire life. How can this be? Easy; you've realized that the buzz of activity around you means that you have survived your operation and entered the recovery phase. You've "made it" through surgery, as the overwhelmingly vast majority of patients do. Although you were fairly certain that the surgery would go smoothly, you were also aware of the risks and afraid of the unknown. Awakening in the recovery room is proof that the unknown is over; you are back in the "real world."

The recovery room is a specialized type of intensive care unit. After surgery, patients are taken there and closely watched for a few hours. The recovery room staff records the patient's vital signs (blood pressure, pulse, respiration), and before patients can be transferred to their room or to an ambulatory discharge area, vital signs must be stable and there must be no evidence of bleeding.

It is not unusual for recovery room patients to have difficulty figuring out the tumult going on around them. An array of nurses seem to be doing all sorts of things simultaneously. One is taking blood pressure, while others are tending to an assortment of instruments with colorful displays and monitors that are beeping and clanging away. (See Chapter 19, "Lines, Bells, and Whistles.")

The most common lines and monitors used in a recovery room are listed below.

LINES AND MONITORS OF THE RECOVERY ROOM

Intravenous lines
Electrocardiograms
Blood pressure cuffs
Pulse oximeter
Drains
Catheters

You still have the intravenous line that was started in the operating room, and you are hooked up to an electrocardiogram (EKG) that records the heart's rate (number of beats per minute) and rhythm.

Your blood pressure may be taken manually or with an automatic blood-pressure monitor, or sphygmomanometer, which checks blood pressure at predetermined intervals.

The pulse oximeter is a relatively new monitor that is very important in the postoperative period because it reflects the cardiovascular and respiratory systems' overall functioning. Through a simple "sensor" that attaches to a finger, toe, or earlobe, the machine measures the oxygen saturation of the blood, and tells the doctors and nurses how well the red blood cells in the lungs are picking up oxygen.

Depending on the extent of your surgery, you may also have a foley catheter in your bladder to measure the kidneys' urine production, and an arterial line that keeps an instant and continuous record of blood pressure. Unlike the automatic blood pressure monitor mentioned above, the arterial line is invasive, gives continuous information, and provides an instant means of drawing blood. The arterial line, like any invasive instrument, presents some risks, such as infection, but this is rare. The arterial line's most severe risk—fortunately, also rare—is interference with the blood supply to the hand by an arterial line in a radial artery. The hand becomes cold and turns white. Fortunately, most people have two main arteries supplying the hand; even if the radial artery is totally occluded, the ulnar artery can easily carry the load. If the ulner artery is not present or is damaged, and the radial artery is occluded by the catheter, the hand can suffer severe and permanent damage, but this scenario is extremely rare.

Although the drain is the one line that is unique to patients undergoing a surgical procedure, not all patients require one. A drain is a tube that is usually connected to a collecting bag or suction apparatus. Its purpose is to remove blood and other fluids from the operative site. Not all patients who have surgery have a drain, but some may have two or more drains, depending on the extensiveness of their surgery.

While lack of privacy is a concern of some patients in intensive care units (see Chapter 20, "The Intensive Care Unit"), this is less of an issue in the recovery room. Here, patients do not have to be bathed, have less of a need to perform private bodily functions, and are typically so groggy that they tend not to think about the other patients around them (who are just as groggy themselves).

What can I do to help in the recovery room?

Do *nothing*! The best thing you can do is to be totally passive. Let the staff do their job, and you "go with the flow." You are most likely still somewhat sedated from the medications administered by the anesthetist during surgery. Anesthesia and sedation interfere with your ability to make a rational decision, and also blur most of your memory of the time you spend in the recovery room. Even when your surgeon visits you in the recovery room, the chances are good that you will not remember his or her visit or instructions. That's why, if you are an ambulatory patient, it is important to go over your instructions for home care with your surgeon before surgery. (See Tips for Ambulatory Patients, right.)

There is only one thing you should have to discuss with the recovery room staff: pain, nausea, or other significant distress such as shortness of breath or chest pain. Nausea and excessive sedation are the most common adverse reactions to anesthesia. Otherwise, it is best to lie quietly and rest.

May I have visitors in the recovery room?

The answer is usually no. Your stay in the recovery room is short. You probably would not remember any visitors anyway, and you certainly don't feel sociable. It's better to concentrate on resting, not on relating to visitors. In addition, the nurses and other staff are very busy, and visitors could interfere with patient care. Finally, not only may the presence of visitors be disturbing to other patients, but the visitors may feel upset by the recovery room's unfamiliar sights and sounds.

There are usually only two exceptions to the no-visitors rule. Parents of small children are often allowed to visit, since their presence may be deeply comforting and reassuring to the child—and they themselves are reassured to see their child safe. And in rare situations, when adult patients have to stay in a recovery room for a long period of time, close family members may be allowed in.

TIPS FOR AMBULATORY PATIENTS

Ambulatory patients who have gone home may still have to deal with the two most common problems that patients face in a recovery room: pain and nausea. So plan ahead. Several days before surgery, ask your surgeon for the prescriptions for analgesics (pain medication) and perhaps antiemetics (medications to control nausea). That way, you can fill your prescriptions before you go to the hospital and have everything you may need ready by your bedside at home.

You may also wish to ask your surgeon and anesthetist for information about the medications you will receive in the recovery room.

How long can I expect to stay in the recovery room?

The rule of thumb is that a patient's time in the recovery room is one to two times the duration of the anesthesia. For example, if your gallbladder operation took an hour, you may expect to be in the recovery room for one to two hours. This is not a hard-and-fast rule, and is clearly affected by how the patient is doing. The duration of anesthesia is, of course, longer than the duration of the operation, since it includes pre- and postsurgery time.

A longer stay in the recovery room doesn't necessarily mean that you are doing poorly. Some people are more sensitive to anesthesia and take longer to wake up or to become alert. A long stay may also stem from extraneous factors. At change of shift, nurses going off duty are busy giving reports on the patients to those coming on duty. During evening shifts, there are often fewer people on the transportation crew. Your assigned bed may not yet have been vacated or cleaned by housekeeping.

The recovery room is a crucial aspect of postoperative care, but it is probably best when you cannot remember it at all. That means that you were well cared-for and did not have to spend enough time there to let it make an impression on you.

DISCHARGE SUMMARY

Admission Date: _____ A.M. P.M.

Discharge Date: _____ A.M. P.M.

IF NO PLATE, PRINT NAME, SEX & HISTORY NO.

Attending Physician: _____ M.D.

DISCHARGE DIAGNOSES **(List in Order of Cause for Hospitalization)** **(Include Comorbidities and Complications)** **Do Not Abbreviate**	**PROCEDURES** **(Include invasive & Non-Invasive** **Procedures)** **Do Not Abbreviate**

_____ DATE: _____

_____ DATE: _____

_____ DATE: _____

_____ DATE: _____

_____ DATE: _____

CHIEF COMPLAINT/REASON FOR ADMISSION: _____

HISTORY OF PRESENT ILLNESS: _____

PHYSICAL EXAMINATION (Pertinent Findings): _____

CHAPTER 19

LINES, BELLS, AND WHISTLES

Machines and devices, wires and tubes, lines and fluids, monitors that beep throughout the night. These crucial components of the hospital armamentarium can seem as intimidating as they are valuable. What *are* all these things? Why are they used and what do they do?

LINES

When physicians and nurses speak about inserting a "line," they are referring to a tube or wire that enters your body through a natural opening, or "port," or through an opening that is specially created for the occasion (such as a puncture of a vein with a needle or an incision through the skin). Tubes and wires are used to monitor, record, measure, control, and/or deliver. Bodily functions that can be measured include temperature, blood pressure, heart rate, output of the kidney and the heart, cardiac and respiratory rhythms, flow of blood and urine, and oxygen concentrations. Certain bodily functions can be controlled by using a line to administer a drug or an electric current, or to deliver a gas such as oxygen.

SOME TYPES OF LINES

In a blood vessel

intravenous

arterial

central

In an organ

foley

nasogastric tube (NG)

Attached to the skin

EKG

Pulse oximeter

Of course, no device is any good by itself; it needs a human being to pay attention to it. Physicians and nurses can't always keep an uninterrupted watch over lines, so they need to be reminded and warned if something is amiss. That's where bells and whistles come into play. Most lines that measure anything are attached to a monitor that measures fluctuations in electrical current, in the degree of pressure through a column of fluid, in the composition of a gas, or in the wavelength of light. The monitors are programmed by specialists to accept certain parameters as normal. Any deviation from these preprogrammed limits sets off an alarm, which can be either visual (flashing lights) or auditory (loud bells and whistles). Whether in intensive care units, operating rooms, or recovery rooms, these alarms can frighten, startle, or confuse patients and family members. They may wonder whether the alarms signify a serious or life-threatening problem—or just a mild irregularity that is not very significant. And frequently when monitors go off, it is a false alarm. Patients and families should be assured that nurses respond to every alarm and will take appropriate steps.

INTRAVENOUS (IV) LINES

The most common lines are those that enter a blood vessel—an artery or a vein. Most common are intravenous lines (those that enter a vein). Patients in intensive care units are often NPO (allowed to ingest nothing by mouth). In order to replace the fluid that the body loses through respiration, sweating, urine, and stool, intravenous fluids such as normal saline, D5W (5 percent dextrose or sugar in water), or Ringer's lactate may be given.

Intravenous lines are fairly safe (though not risk-free), and have many uses. IV lines are used to administer such fluids as medication, saline, sugar water, or blood when a person cannot or should not be given fluids by mouth; a person cannot safely swallow; speed is of the essence; or fluids must directly enter the bloodstream.

An intravenous line can be placed into a vein anywhere in the body. Most commonly, IVs are placed in the arm or hand because they are better tolerated by the patient, are more readily accessible, and carry a lower incidence of complications than other sites.

To locate a suitable vein, a tourniquet is tied around the desired area. This causes veins to engorge so that they can be seen or felt. Once the IV is inserted through the skin and into the middle of the vein, blood will suddenly appear in the thin tubing attached to it, indicating that the IV has successfully penetrated the vein.

The insertion of the intravenous line is definitely the worst part of the experience, because veins and skin can be quite sensitive. Anesthesia usually is not used because arteries and veins cannot be anesthetized reliably or easily with local anesthesia. Furthermore, the discomfort of having the IV inserted is transient and the needle can be left in place without continuing pain. At times, especially when one is about to undergo surgery, the physician injects a small amount of local anesthesia directly into the skin, creating a small bump resembling a mosquito bite or bee sting; the bump is called a wheal.

Once the IV is inserted, it is attached to an inverted tube, bottle, or bag of fluid. Great care is taken to keep the entire system as sterile as possible, because the IV site can be a potential entryway for germs into the body. Gauze pads and tape are used to anchor the IV safely to the right spot.

The part of the intravenous line that actually penetrates the vein is either a catheter or a butterfly needle. An intravenous catheter is a plastic tube that enters the vein through a hole in the wall of the vein. A butterfly needle is a hollow metal tube with two plastic wings (resembling those on a butterfly) that are used to manipulate the needle during insertion and to hold it in place. Intravenous catheters are more stable and more difficult to dislodge because they occupy a greater length of the vein. They are more difficult to insert, however, and more likely to cause a complication.

Arterial lines, which are placed within an artery, are less frequently used because the insertion procedure is more complicated, painful, and risky; if infection or thrombosis (clotting of the artery) occurs, the circulation to an entire extremity can be jeopardized.

TKO LINES

Although most IV lines are always left attached to the source of fluid, a "TKO" IV line is not attached to anything. TKO stands for "to keep open." With most intravenous lines, the IV fluid is continually dripping into the vein and, therefore, the patient's IV is attached to a bag what hangs from a pole. This interferes with use of the hand and with ambulation. If the patient does not require continuous administration of IV fluids and only the intermittent administration of medication (such as antibiotics), then a

> ### TYPES OF INTRAVENOUS FLUIDS
>
> **Ringer's lactate**
> **Normal saline**
> **D5W**
> **Combinations of the above**
> **Albumisol**
> **Plasma**
> **Blood:**
> **Whole blood**
> **Packed cells**
> **Blood factors**
> **Platelets**

TKO line may be used. It is not attached to a bag, so a patient can use the hand and walk without such restrictions.

Thus, a TKO line is a "placeholder" that keeps a vein accessible. This is done for two reasons. Most commonly, the patient requires medication to be given intravenously every few hours, but does not require intravenous fluids continuously. It is, therefore, more convenient for the patient to have a TKO line instead of being tethered to a fluid source. The other instance a TKO is used is when doctors are concerned about your medical condition and decide to leave the line in place in case of an emergency.

COMPLICATIONS ASSOCIATED WITH IV LINES

Most hospitals have teams of professionals or technicians who are trained and skilled in the insertion of intravenous lines. A good rule of thumb is: No matter what a person's position or rank in the medical hierarchy, if he or she misses your vein twice, ask for someone else to try again.

Once an IV line is placed, it should not routinely hurt. If you have discomfort, call the nurse to have the site of the intravenous line evaluated.

WORRIES ABOUT BUBBLES AND BLOOD

Many people have heard stories about patients dying as a result of bubbles in intravenous line tubing that enter a vein. However, this is a highly exaggerated concern. It takes a huge amount of air, injected with some force, to cause harm. Hence, seeing a bubble or two in the intravenous tubing should not be cause for alarm.

Similarly, you needn't worry about air bubbles if your IV bottle has become empty. Since there is no fluid pushing the air in, it is more likely that your blood will actually back up into the IV tubing. This stains the tubing red and can seem very scary. But it is unlikely to be dangerous. If the blood remains in the tubing long enough, it will clot and the IV will then need to be replaced. If there is only staining in the tubing, it is of no concern.

Of course, if you have any concern that an intravenous line may be malfunctioning, inform your nurse or physician.

Complications include the following:

Sensitivity to medication. Some medications, such as certain antibiotics and many chemotherapeutic agents, can cause irritation. In some instances, doctors can substitute less irritating intravenous medications. Other options are to make the medication more dilute, or to give it more slowly, or to use a line placed in a larger vein.

Extravasation. In this condition, the medication or other fluid that is supposedly flowing through the tubing and into your blood vessel is not staying within your vein. Fluid may be leaking around the catheter or through a hole in the vein into the surrounding space (subcutaneous tissues). Some medications can be quite damaging to the tissue. In certain clinical situations, such as chemotherapy administration, this occurs rather often and is an unfortunate but unavoidable risk. One recourse is to inject steroids into the site or to apply iced compresses.

Infection. Infection is always a concern when the skin is penetrated; an IV site must be kept free of bacteria that can cause infection when IV sites are left for long periods of time. In some instances, a person may be especially vulnerable to infection. For example, patients who are receiving chemotherapy through a central venous line are more prone to infection because of decreases in their white blood cell count.

Phlebitis. Intravenous lines should not be left in any single spot for more than approximately forty-eight hours, depending on the clinical situation. Lines that are left in too long can cause phlebitis, an inflammation of the vein. Phlebitis may occur in reaction to the catheter, to the medication, or to infection.

If you are having pain at an IV site or notice any redness, tell your doctor or nurse. When phlebitis does occur in a vein in the hand or arm, although uncomfortable and temporarily traumatic to that section of vein, it usually does not cause long-term problems or complications. If nurses don't seem to keep track of IVs, you can do so yourself by writing (on the tape holding it in place) the time and day an intravenous line was placed. This provides a gentle reminder to the staff and makes you feel more confident that the IV site will be changed when necessary.

WARNING SIGNS OF PHLEBITIS

Pain
Swelling
Redness
Warmth

IV FLUIDS

The types of fluids that flow through an intravenous line are numerous and vary according to the patient's condition. Among the most commonly used fluids are:

Ringer's lactate. This solution contains sterile water, salts, and minerals intended to match the composition of your body fluids.

Normal saline (NS). A solution of sterile water and sodium chloride (salt) used to replace your fluid needs (water), it keeps the concentration of all types of salts in your body and blood constant (isotonic).

D5W. This solution is 5 percent dextrose in water.

Albumisol or plasmanate. Water and proteins naturally found in your blood make up this solution, but in a more dilute concentration.

Plasma. This fluid is blood without the cellular elements. At one time, lost blood could only be replaced with whole blood (blood taken from the vein of a donor, tested, then given unchanged into the patient). Then techniques evolved that could separate plasma from cells so that just the cells are given back. Patients in a fragile medical state may need the red blood cells but not necessarily all the other components that would add volume to the transfusion and might upset the patient's circulatory system. Now techniques have become so sophisticated that individual types of cells can be separated and given back as needed. For example, patients may be given platelets if they are bleeding due to a low platelet count (thrombocytopenia), or white blood cells if theirs are low in number or are not working properly.

LONG-TERM IV USE

Many forms of intravenous therapy that once would have required long-term hospitalization or multiple punctures for new intravenous lines can now be safely done on an outpatient basis, or even in the patient's own home or place of employment. Such types of therapy include antibiotic therapy for osteomyelitis (bone infection) and endocarditis (infection of the lining of the heart). If people need intravenous antibiotics, usually a visiting nurse service will come to the patient's home or office three or four times a day to administer them through a chronic indwelling catheter that may be totally under the skin, or may exit at some place through the skin of the neck or upper chest. (The visiting nurse service is ordered by the physician; however, not all health insurance plans cover it.)

Another type of situation requiring long-term (six- to twelve-month) intravenous therapy is chemotherapy for cancer. Sufficient intravenous access can be a problem; doctors and nurses may not be able to find enough veins that can accommodate a butterfly or intravenous catheter. Patients who receive long-term chemotherapy or who have been in the hospital for a long time are often said to have "used up their veins," meaning that it is hard to find a valid IV site. This problem occurs because drugs that go into the veins can damage the vein walls, causing the veins to sclerose (close down due to inflammation and scarring) so that no blood can flow through them.

The solution is to create access to large veins, which are more resistant to sclerosis. Through a very minor surgical procedure, a doctor—usually a surgeon or anesthesiologist—places a long-term indwelling catheter into a large vein. One of the most common is the Broviac catheter. The superficial end of the catheter, which can be just under or just above the skin, has a port attached to it. The medical staff gives medication by placing a needle into the port. If the port is beneath the skin, the needle is placed through the skin and then into the port. The other end of the catheter travels from the port through the tissues under the skin (fat, muscle, etc.) and into a larger vein. From here it travels down toward the heart. It ends just above the heart in the superior vena cava, which is one of the two large veins that empty all the blood returning from the body into the heart. The advantage of this is that the catheter is in a large vein with lots of blood flow so that the problems of phlebitis from the catheter and medication are essentially eliminated.

The main risk is that of infection through the skin, either because the catheter passes through the skin or because the needle passes through the skin into the port. In the former case, the dressing around the catheter must be kept meticulously clean and changed in a precise sterile fashion. This can be done by the patient or a family member, but usually is best done by whatever service comes to the patient's home or office to administer the medication. In the latter case, the skin must be thoroughly prepped prior to introducing the needle into the port through the skin.

"BELLS AND WHISTLES": THE FUNCTIONAL MUSIC OF MONITORS

A MEDLEY OF MONITORS

Imagine giving a nursery school class an assortment of noisemakers and toy musical instruments to play all at once. The resulting cacophony resembles the percussive background noise to which patients on monitors in intensive care units and recovery rooms are exposed twenty-four hours a day—but with one important difference: There's nothing random about these beeps and bells, whistles and blips, chimes and buzzers. Every sound represents a meaningful measure being taken by a medical device called a monitor; some patients may have many different monitors at once.

Monitors are devices that *detect* and *communicate* information about how a patient's body is functioning. Since they are attached to a patient's body, either briefly or for an extended period of time, they can serve as additional "eyes and ears and fingers" for the medical staff. Although some patients feel that monitors are intimidating, even "cold," they are potentially lifesaving machines that represent significant advances in medical technology.

Some commonly used monitors include:

Blood Pressure (BP) monitor. This records the systolic and diastolic blood pressures. Blood pressure results are given as a ratio, e.g., 120 over 80, or 120/80. The systolic blood pressure is the upper number (120), and refers to the rhythmically recurrent *contractions* of the heart when it pumps out blood; the diastolic blood pressure is the lower number (80) and refers to the rhythmically recurrent *expansions* of the cavities of the heart when they fill with blood.

Electrocardiogram (EKG). A monitor that measures the rate and rhythm of the heart.

Expiratory Gas Monitor. This records the gases in the air exhaled from the lungs and helps make sure that for a patient on a respirator, the placement of the endotracheal tube is correct.

Intravenous Pump. A monitor that assures that the regulated fluids are going into the patient through the intravenous line at the proper rate. Also called a "Harvard pump."

Pulse Oximeter. This measures both the oxygen saturation of the blood and the heart rate.

Respiratory Rate Monitor. A device that records the rhythm of breathing and the number of times per minute the patient is breathing.

How Monitors Work

Monitors all appear and function differently, but they have one common purpose: to alert the medical staff if any problem has occurred. Monitors "notify" the staff in two ways: aurally, by sounding a bell or alarm, and visually, through a display where data can be seen. There are two types of displays:

Graphic displays. For example, a wave that undulates across the screen, such as an electrocardiogram (EKG), which has a graphic display that records the heart rate and the pattern of the heart muscle's normal or abnormal contractions.

Digital displays. A display of numbers; for example, a pulse oximeter has a digital display that shows the measured oxygen in the blood. Other types of digital displays show parameters, or ranges, of numbers that doctors or nurses have entered into the monitor. A Harvard pump, for example, may have a range of numbers for pressure in the intravenous line and the rate at which fluid is passing through the IV. If the pressure becomes too high and/or the fluid rate too low, the monitor sounds.

The bell/alarm and the display reflect data collected by the *sensor*— the part of the monitor that attaches to the patient's body and "senses" specific functions. In an EKG, for example, the sensor is usually a group of four to five electrodes that are sticky and placed on the patient's skin in a particular pattern. The sensor on a pulse oximeter is a clip with a light in it that is attached to a finger, toe, or even an earlobe.

Some sensors may be attached to a line. For example, the sensor on a respirator monitor is in the "circuit" to which the endotracheal tube is attached. The sensor determines that the endotracheal tube is attached properly and that the respiratory rate is uniform and within the preestablished limits.

As helpful as monitors can be, they also have a down side: Often the alarms they sound are really *false* alarms that needlessly frighten patients or visitors. Don't allow the alarms to alarm you; the staff can tell when a monitor is just "acting up," and when its alarm is a bona fide alert.

CHAPTER 20

THE INTENSIVE CARE UNIT

Intensive care—a consistent and focused level of observation, monitoring, and attention for people in critical need—is one of a hospital's most valuable and life-saving services. Being admitted to an intensive care unit may be a worrisome sign that one's condition may be critical, but patients and their families can also be reassured and relieved that they are getting the closest attention hospitals have to offer.

Many people don't realize that the value of intensive care units, or ICUs, was not really recognized until the 1950s, when studies revealed that hospitalized heart attack patients who received intensive care had a higher chance of survival than those on a regular medical floor. Before long, physicians from other specialties demanded intensive care for their patients as well. Not only did patients receive better care and prove more likely to recover, but problems previously considered insoluble, such as septic shock and pulmonary failure, now became treatable.

Today, there are so many different intensive care units that they begin to sound like alphabet soup: SICU, CCU, MICU, SDU, NICU, PICU—and the list is still growing.

The changing physical plant of the world-renowned New York Hospital illustrates the proliferation of intensive care units. When the hospital was built in 1923, it did not have a single bed in an intensive care unit. But when its new facility, the New York Hospital–Cornell Medical Center, opens at the dawn of the twenty-first century, fully 60 percent of the beds will be allocated to intensive care.

TYPES OF INTENSIVE CARE UNITS

CCU: Coronary Care Unit (for disorders of the heart)
MICU: Medical Intensive Care Unit (for noncardiac internal medicine problems)
NICU: Neonatal Intensive Care Unit (for newborn babies)
PICU: Pulmonary Intensive Care Unit (for disorders of the heart and lungs)
SICU: Surgical Intensive Care Unit (for postsurgery and massive trauma such as burns)
SDU: Step Down Unit (an intermediate unit between a full-blown ICU and the floor)

THE UNIQUE FEATURES OF INTENSIVE CARE

What makes a room an intensive care unit is not only sophisticated equipment and monitors, but also the nurses' and doctors' high degree of specialization and experience. ICU nurses, among the elite of their profession, are trained to recognize emergencies quickly and to initiate emergency care and patient support while a physician is being summoned.

Intensive care units also have a much higher ratio of nurses to patients. A typical medical floor of thirty to forty patients may have five nurses (one head nurse and four staff nurses) during the day and perhaps two nurses at night. In an intensive care unit, the ratio of nurses to patients is one-to-one or one-to-two during all shifts, so nurses can pay more attention to their patients and respond rapidly if problems occur.

The time it takes for a doctor to respond to the call of an ICU nurse is usually quite short. In most ICUs, a physician is present at all times, often even eating and sleeping there. Despite the exhausting schedule, interns and residents in teaching institutions often cite the ICU as their favorite rotation. Here they feel on the cutting edge of medicine, and savor a great feeling of accomplishment as they help save the life of a critically ill adult, child, or infant. Some of these young physicians and surgeons go on to become "intensivists," specialists in the care of critically ill patients. They may not have a private practice, and you may not remember their name (or recognize it when you get their bill), but they can play a major role in saving your life.

WHY PATIENTS ARE SENT TO INTENSIVE CARE UNITS

Being placed in an intensive care unit is not necessarily an indication that a patient is truly in critical condition, but rather that he or she needs very close attention. Intensive care is routine for after-care following some surgical procedures (such as repair of an aortic aneurysm), for certain diagnostic issues such as the need to rule out a heart attack after chest pain, or for monitoring a patient who has suffered major trauma or burns.

In nonroutine cases, admission to the ICU may indicate serious problems or just a temporary setback on the road to recovery: A patient who cannot breathe needs a tube inserted into the trachea so that oxygen can reach the lungs; a postoperative patient who is bleeding excessively needs more intravenous fluids or a blood transfusion; a bleeding patient may need to be returned to the operating room for control of the bleeding, or may have another medical problem that must be attended to before the bleeding will stop; a cardiac patient with a life-threatening heart rhythm abnormality needs to have the heart rhythm restored to normal.

Among the most common reasons for admission to an ICU are:

Heart attack (myocardial infarction). Also, if there are changes in the rate or rhythm of the heart (arrhythmia, tachycardia, bradycardia).

Sudden, excessive bleeding. This might occur either after surgery or from such conditions as an acute flare-up of a bleeding ulcer.

Infection (sepsis, gram-negative sepsis, septic shock). Certain virulent germs or bacteria, such as in an abscess or the blood stream, cause the heart, lungs, liver, and/or kidneys to malfunction. Blood pressure gets too low, the kidneys do not make enough urine, and the lungs cannot deliver enough oxygen to the blood.

**TEN MOST COMMON
REASONS FOR ADMISSION
TO AN ICU**

Angina (chest pain)
**Myocardial infarction
(heart attack)**
**Apnea/respiratory arrest
(difficulty breathing)**
**Arrhythmia
(abnormal heart rhythm)**
Burn
**Hemorrhage
(severe bleeding)**
**Hypotension
(low blood pressure)**
**Monitoring sepsis
(blood poisoning)**
Stroke
Trauma (severe accident)

Abnormally low blood pressure (hypotension). This might be caused by any of the above conditions. The definition of "abnormal" varies from person to person. In a person who usually has high blood pressure and normally runs a systolic pressure (the first number in the blood pressure) of 150, a pressure of 80 would be low. However, in a person who normally has a systolic blood pressure of 90, a systolic pressure of 80 is fine. When a person's blood pressure is too low compared to what the vital organs (heart, kidneys, liver, brain) are used to, these organs do not perform normally. When a patient is admitted to an intensive care unit for hypotension the first thing doctors look for is a heart problem, bleeding, or infection, all of which can lead to shock by causing low blood pressure.

Severe trauma. When trauma is so severe that life support and monitoring are required. Trauma may be associated with the severe stress or abnormal conditions of a long and serious surgical procedure; injury caused by such catastrophic events as a motor vehicle accident, a fire, or a severe farm or industrial accident; or such violence as beatings, gunshots, or knife wounds.

How sick is a patient in the ICU? Don't count on getting the answer from the hospital operator. Generally, when people are in intensive care and you call the hospital to find out how they are, you are told that they are "on the critical list." This sounds ominous, but frequently, patients are only being monitored for their protection and are not truly critically ill. In fact, not only is there not any actual "list," but you are speaking to an operator who has never seen the patient in question, and has been trained to respond with that phrase to all queries about ICU patients. Even if a patient is doing fine and is just waiting in the intensive care unit until an appropriate bed on the floor becomes available, the hospital would still consider that patient on the critical list until the move to the floor has taken place. To find out how someone in an intensive care unit is really doing, ask the physician or nurse. Patients always have the right to request that doctors and nurses refrain from giving out such information.

MOST COMMON MONITORS USED IN AN ICU

EKG: Electrocardiogram measures heart rate and rhythm.
Pulse oximeter: Measures the amount of oxygen in the red blood cells.
BP monitor: Automatically measures and records the blood pressure.
Transducers: Measures pressure in a line and translates it into numbers for display.
RR monitor: Measures respiratory rate; how many times per minute the patient breathes.

THE ICU EXPERIENCE

A PLETHORA OF TECHNOLOGIES

You are lying in a hospital bed, attached to a variety of tubes, lines, and wires, which may include one or more of the following:

Intravenous line (IV). In your arm, leg, or neck; a neck IV is probably the most uncomfortable and awkward, since it can be hard to turn your head. Its use may indicate that other, more accessible veins were not good enough to use.

Endotracheal tube. In your mouth or nose if you are having respiratory problems, the endotracheal tube is hooked to the respirator, which breathes for you until you can breathe again on your own.

Electrocardiogram pads. Attached to your chest, arms, and back to monitor your heart rate.

**MOST COMMON "LINES"
USED IN AN ICU**

Intravenous line or IV

Arterial or radial line

Venous lines:
CVP
   Swan-Ganz
   Subclavian
   Internal jugular
   External jugular

Cutdown
   (arterial or venous line
   not accessed with a
   needle stick)

Foley catheter
   (tube placed to drain and
   measure urine)

Chest tube
   (tube placed to either
   drain chest cavity or keep
   lungs inflated)

Surgical drains

Nasogastric tube
   (tube placed to drain
   stomach)

Endotracheal tube

Clip or electrode. Attached to your finger, toe, or earlobe (pulse oximeter) to measure the oxygen saturation of your blood (Sa02). The highest level is 100; doctors and nurses like to see it in the 90s if possible.

Arm cuff. To measure your blood pressure at regular intervals, the arm cuff may be annoying, as it is set to measure your blood pressure automatically every five to ten minutes, a sensation like an iron grip on your biceps.

Catheter. A tube going through your urethra into your bladder, so you don't have to worry about getting up to go to the bathroom to void (urinate).

Other lines. For example, a radial line that goes into your artery continually measures your blood pressure; or a line inserted into a deeper and more centrally located vein (central line, subclavian line, an internal or external jugular line, swan ganz line) that can continually measure venous pressures, or even the pressures in your heart if you are more critically ill. (See Chapter 19, "Lines, Bells, and Whistles.")

AN IMPERSONAL EXCELLENCE

In many intensive care units, especially in older hospitals, there is no such thing as your own space. There is probably no wall between you and the patients to your left and right; in fact, they may be just two or three arms' lengths away from you. A curtain is usually available for privacy if somebody remembers to pull it. In any event, you probably will never see your "neighbors" again after you are discharged from the hospital—and if you are sick enough to require a stay in the intensive care unit, privacy may be the last thing you're worried about.

Sometimes ICU patients or their families feel that they have no control over what happens to them in the unit. Although care is excellent, it may not necessarily feel "personalized": ICU physicians and nurses do not have much time to focus on patients' material comforts because they are so busy paying attention to their critical medical needs.

Many ICU staff also develop a certain self-protective shell. If they do not get too attached to their seriously ill patients, then they will not be so upset if patients do not have good outcomes. This protective mechanism functions most consistently for patients who are in the ICU for short periods of time. But when patients are in the ICU for weeks and months, the barrier tends to break down. The doctors and the nurses become so emotionally attached that a death affects them almost as much as a family member. In pediatric intensive care units, this is especially intense. The patients are usually there for longer periods of time, so there is greater opportunity to develop emotional attachments. Additionally, many physicians and nurses find it much more difficult to accept and handle the loss of an infant or a child than an adult. Because of the grief associated with intensive care, emotional burnout is an occupational hazard and ICU nursing staff tends to have high turnover.

The ICU Schedule

An intensive care unit has no day and no night. The following schedule, therefore, is somewhat arbitrary. Motion, attention, and action are constants in the ICU, where every moment presents the potential for emergency.

5:00 A.M. The intensive care unit nurse who is scheduled to finish her shift in a couple of hours gets geared up now so that you will be all clean and fresh to face a new day. To start with, if you managed to fall asleep at about 3:00 a.m., nurses awaken you, change your sheets, and bathe you. They also do your "line care." For example, if you have a large catheter going into one of the larger veins in your body (a central line), the spot where the catheter punctures the skin must be cleansed with an antiseptic solution, then rebandaged in a sterile fashion so as to combat infection.

6:00 A.M. A bedraggled house officer comes in to draw your blood and take a quick look at you before formal morning rounds to make sure everything seems all right.

7:00 A.M. Morning house-staff rounds begin. The house officer you saw an hour ago now appears with a gang of more senior house officers (residents) and medical students to poke you more. Their jargon-ridden conversations may seem to be in a foreign language—and it can be disconcerting to realize they are talking about you, perhaps without seeking your participation or input. Many patients are afraid to ask questions at this point. Although these busy interns and residents do not have a great deal of time to answer your questions, if you are concerned or even frightened by what you hear, you certainly are entitled to ask questions to put your mind at ease.

8:00 A.M. Breakfast. Sorry, no pancakes if you're NPO (allowed to have nothing by mouth), or have a tube down your throat that makes it somewhat difficult to eat. Nutrition is very important to your recovery, and most ICUs have a nutritionist on staff, but your nutritional needs may be met via IV or tube.

In many intensive care units, if you are well enough to sit up and feed yourself a full breakfast, you are probably about to be transferred out of the unit. In such units as the CCU (coronary care unit), most patients are there only for monitoring purposes and are usually given regular food that conforms to a low-fat, low-salt, no-sugar diet.

9:00 A.M. Time for rounds again. The same people who were there at 6:00 A.M. and 7:00 A.M. return with more doctors who are this time wearing longer white coats. These are the intensive care unit attending physicians. The rounds usually also include representatives from the other professional staffs (e.g., nurses, therapists, etc.). They review any changes in your condition over the last twenty-four hours and plan your treatment for the next twenty-four hours.

Sometime in the interval between 6:00 A.M. and 9:00 A.M., your private attending physician and the house staff from his or her service will also come in to check on you and confer on your care in a round of their own.

For the next six hours or so (until about 3:00 P.M.), the decisions made during rounds will be enacted. You may, for example, need a chest X ray or an electrocardiogram, and need to have more blood drawn. You may get physical therapy, such as chest PT (the therapist pounds on your chest, encourages you to cough and breathe deeply) to make sure that your lungs stay clear and no problems such as pneumonia develop. The schedule of these activities is such that if you were planning on getting any sleep during the day, forget it!

12 NOON. Lunch: See breakfast.

4:00 P.M. Afternoon rounds. The exact time may vary, but presuming that you are stable and improving, this is the next time that you will see some of your doctors. They will recapitulate the results of the day's tests and identify trends in your vital signs (temperature, heart rate, blood pressure, etc.). Any tests that cannot wait until after tomorrow's morning rounds will be ordered now and performed during the evening.

5:00 P.M. Dinner: See lunch.

Not much is usually planned for between dinner and five the next morning. Any tests that could not be performed during the day or that were ordered on afternoon rounds will probably be performed at this time. The intensive care unit remains noisy and the lights stay on high, which may make it difficult to get any sleep.

VISITING THE ICU

Visiting hours in intensive care units are always shorter than on regular patient floors. Patients are usually quite ill and should not get overtired from playing host. And there is always a lot of activity going on, so patient families might get in the way. In most intensive care units, visitors are allowed to visit for fifteen minutes at a time between the hours of 6–8 P.M. Some ICUs are more generous, with nurses often allowing a family member in during nonvisiting hours if the patient's condition and the nurses' schedule permit it.

Visiting in the ICU is not for the squeamish or faint at heart. Anything can happen there, including cardiac arrests, bleeding, and worse. Your loved ones can be hooked up to a million different tubes, intravenous lines, and wires, and may be pale, tired, and in pain. What is amazing—and heartening—is how quickly people can return to looking normal as the devices are removed.

A Disorienting Sleeplessness

The ICU's constant activity and bright lights result in severe sleep deprivation for many patients, and especially in some older people, produces a form of agitation known as ICU psychosis. People who may have been brilliant all their lives suddenly lose touch with reality. They may seem disoriented, resisting treatment, seem to lose their memory, become caustic, nasty, or withdrawn. They may jeopardize their treatment by yanking out IV lines or trying to jump out of bed. Such behavior is frightening for both patients and their families, especially if the patients must be physically restrained in the bed to prevent them from pulling out lines or leaving the bed. Nothing is more demeaning than to be put in physical restraints, and it is only done as a last resort to prevent patients from harming themselves or others. Restraints, however, are only the epitome of the loss of control that patients suffer in ICUs, where body functions can be controlled by machines, nurses, or physicians; no wonder some people get so disoriented.

Luckily, ICU psychosis is reversible if patients were normal before and are restored to their usual state of health, and is not a harbinger of approaching senility. The treatment usually consists of transferring the patient to a regular floor if at all medically possible. If not, a family member is usually asked to sit with the patient for extended periods to create a more familiar environment. If all else fails, drugs are administered to calm the patient.

The majority of ICU patients eventually return to normal functioning. Occasionally, however, despite all of the best therapy available, a devastating condition proves irreversible; a brain-dead patient hooked up to all the supporting technology has no hope of recovery. These tragic situations occur commonly and raise many ethical questions. Should this patient get additional therapy? When do we terminate life support? Who makes these decisions?

There are no definitive answers to these questions. Each case is slightly different and must be addressed by family members, the patient's physicians and nurses, chaplains, hospital administrators, and occasionally lawyers—and by patients themselves, who can help avert anguish for their families by writing "living wills" while they are still able to do so. (See Chapter 6, "Patients' Rights.")

CHAPTER 21

OBSTETRICS

Of all departments in the hospital, people are most likely to be happy in obstetrics, where the excruciating intensity of labor culminates in an event of incomparable celebration: the miracle of new life.

Due to the popularity of childbirth education classes, more parents-to-be than ever before are prepared in advance for the hospital experience. These classes, for which women can obtain a referral from their obstetrician or nurse-midwife, explain the process of pregnancy and the importance of prenatal care, and teach breathing techniques, massage, and laboring and birth positions that can help women cope with contractions and maintain stamina and focus throughout the stages of labor. Pregnant women attend the classes with their "labor partner"—the person who will actively participate in supporting them during labor. Usually, the labor partner is the woman's husband, but some women are accompanied by a friend, their mother or sister, or another relative. Labor partners learn how to coach the woman on breathing techniques, to offer massage and encouragement, to provide light nourishment when appropriate, and to communicate with the doctor and nurses.

The most well-known form of childbirth preparation is Lamaze. While Lamaze and other childbirth techniques are primarily intended to enable a woman to experience "natural childbirth" (vaginal delivery without anesthesia), instructors also address the full range of options for pain relief and delivery.

Vaginal delivery is possible in most but not all births. Cesarean-section delivery may be necessary if there are maternal or fetal complications; if there are twins, triplets, or more; if a baby is too large to fit through the birth canal; if a woman has herpes or another condition that could be transmitted to the baby during childbirth; or if labor "fails to progress" and the cervix does not fully dilate (open) despite many hours of contractions.

HOSPITAL TOURS

In addition to childbirth classes, many couples also prepare for their hospital delivery by taking a tour of the delivery and nursery (often both the regular nursery and neonatal intensive care nurseries) weeks or months before the due date.

Many hospitals also have valuable tours for siblings-to-be. Children enjoy feeling included in the process of preparing for the new arrival, and when they return to the hospital to visit after the birth, they are reassured to have some familiarity with the setting. (If your hospital has no regularly scheduled adults' or children's tours, request one.)

LABOR BEGINS

Women who arrive at the hospital feeling ready to give birth are evaluated by physicians and nurses to see if they are, in fact, ready. In some instances, they prove to be in the relatively early stages of labor and are asked to go home and return later, when contractions are closer together and/or the water breaks and/or there are other indications that delivery is imminent.

You may feel very disappointed if "sent away," but you probably will be more comfortable laboring at home—and the hospital staff will have the time and space to devote to other women who are in the later stages of labor. However, if you feel strongly about wanting to remain, speak up. For example, if you have a history of short labors with previous children, or if you live a distance from the hospital and are concerned about the travel, you may be able to stay.

ADMISSION

Once it is determined that you are indeed ready to be admitted, you are taken to the labor floor, and your husband or other labor partner can join you. The "prepping" and procedures from this point on depend in large part on your doctor or nurse-midwife's approach, your own preferences, your condition, and the condition of the fetus(es).

Prepping, a nickname for "preparing," may or may not include shaving the pubic area, taking an enema, having an intravenous line placed as a precaution or for administration of medication or nutrients, and having a maternal monitor placed on your abdomen to monitor the fetus's heartbeat during the stress of delivery. Some doctors use fetal monitors as well. Which prepping and procedures are done, and when, is a matter to discuss in advance with your doctor. Some couples and their doctors prepare a "birth plan" listing their preferences, and send it to the hospital to keep on file. In addition to prepping and procedures, a birth plan also may cover your wishes as to these matters:

- To have your husband, partner, or other individual who attended Lamaze classes stay with you throughout labor and delivery.
- To be in a "birthing room" (a room that resembles a homey bedroom) instead of a standard delivery/operating room, if you have a normal vaginal delivery.
- To breastfeed your newborn exclusively, or to allow limited supplemental formula.
- To have your baby "room in" (stay with you in your room instead of in the nursery, during all or part of your hospital stay).

PAIN CONTROL

Lamaze techniques can truly help a woman cope with labor pains, but natural childbirth is not for everyone. Women have different pain thresholds; even those who may have intended to avoid pain medication may decide to request it if labor is especially difficult or prolonged. Anesthesia done properly will not hurt the baby and doesn't mean that you are a failure or a wimp. Labor is not an endurance test or an indicator of courage. It is a strenuous process for which you should obtain whatever support you need.

If you do decide to have pain medication, the most common route of administration is an epidural catheter placed in your lower back, near (but not in) the spinal column. An epidural numbs you from the waist down, affording you a great deal of pain relief while still enabling you to stay conscious and aware. You can speak with those around you, and—most thrilling of all—you can see your baby's birth and hear his or her first cry.

AFTER THE DELIVERY

As with labor itself, what happens after the birth varies according to the doctor or nurse-midwife, the hospital's policies, the parents' wishes, and the baby's and mother's conditions. You may be able to cuddle your newborn for quite a while after it is born, or the baby may need to be cleaned and examined immediately. Mother and baby may be separated, with the mother taken to her room and the baby to the newborn nursery, or may share a room. Nothing is lovelier than rooming in, but you may feel so exhausted following the birth that you may wish to have the baby cared for in the nursery so you can get some rest. Some women, for example, ask for the baby to spend the first night in the nursery and to be brought to them every couple of hours for breast or bottle feeding. Then the baby rooms in for most or all of the rest of the hospital stay.

Some babies born by cesarean, most premature babies, and any infants with cardiac or other problems are admitted to a neonatal intensive care unit (NICU) for monitoring. The need for monitoring or treatment is sometimes known in advance of birth (for example, if it is clear that a birth is quite premature) but may be determined by a variety of physical findings and reflex tests performed by the doctor on all infants to assess their health and maturity.

CESAREAN DELIVERY

If you have to have a cesarean delivery, you can still have anesthesia via an epidural (unless it's an emergency cesarean that requires general anesthesia), thus enabling you to be awake for the first glimpse of your new son or daughter. You will need to go to a recovery room after the baby and placenta are delivered and the incision is sewn. But you may be able to have your baby stay with you there if your husband or other labor partner is there to help.

A cesarean requires more extensive recuperation time than vaginal delivery, of course, but you can still breastfeed and care for your baby. Some women feel bitterly disappointed that they did not have a vaginal delivery, but it is important to remember that the most important goal of birth is to preserve the mother's and baby's health. Nevertheless, it can be encouraging to know that the phrase "once a cesarean, always a cesarean" does not always hold true. In a subsequent birth, you may be able to have a vaginal delivery, if the reasons that you had a cesarean this time are no longer present.

A few words of advice if you've had a cesarean:

- Try to get up and walking as soon as your doctor advises. You may feel that it's impossible to stand up straight and take a step, but be assured that your stitches won't come out and your recuperation will proceed more smoothly the sooner you're up and around.
- At the same time, don't *rush* your recuperation. Sit up in bed, start walking, but don't try to be a hero. Let people help you. If it's a strain to reach for the phone, take it off the hook or let someone else answer. If visitors are too much of a strain, ask them to wait until you've been home a few weeks before they stop by.
- When you hold or feed your baby, place a pillow across your abdomen to protect your incision. Newborns may look fragile, but it's amazing how powerfully they can kick!

LENGTH OF HOSPITAL STAY

If you had natural childbirth and have been brought to your room to recover, don't get too comfortable. The government and the health insurance industry seek to have mother and child discharged as quickly as possible after a normal vaginal delivery—perhaps even on the same day.

The hurry to discharge new mothers is unfortunate. Whether you've had a vaginal or cesarean delivery, you need rest to recuperate from the exhausting experience of labor and childbirth; to cope with the physical, hormonal, and emotional postpartum changes; and to help breastfeeding get off to a good start. Once you go home, you may not be able to get the rest you need if you have other children and household matters to take care of, as well as the newborn. Furthermore, in-hospital classes on how to care for, bathe, and breastfeed your baby are traditionally offered during the three or four hospital days after delivery. If you're a first-time parent, these classes are great opportunities to learn the basics of baby care.

GETTING HELP AT HOME

After any hospital stay, it's a good idea to arrange for someone to help you when you go home—and after you've had a baby, it's essential. Have your husband take paternity leave; your parents or in-laws visit for a week or two; ask several friends to pitch in; or hire a baby nurse or a doula (a person who assists new mothers at home). That way, someone other than you can help care for other children, prepare meals, do laundry, answer the phone, greet visitors, write thank-you notes for baby gifts, organize the nursery, and deal with other household responsibilities—thereby freeing you to rest and get breastfeeding established. It is astonishing how much time and energy are required in caring for a tiny baby—and you need someone to take care of you, too, during your recovery and adjustment to new parenthood.

CHAPTER 22

HEALING AT HOME: CONVALESCENCE AND HOME-CARE SERVICES

Twenty years ago, patients who felt they needed a few more days to convalesce in the hospital could simply ask their attending physician to extend their stay. Someone who lived alone, for example, might explain that he could not afford to hire a nurse or nurse's aide to look after him. A busy parent might explain that her only chance for rest was in the hospital; once home, her children would clamor for attention and she would have scant chance to lie still and let healing take its course. Doctors usually assumed that since nobody particularly likes being in the hospital, patients who wanted to stay had valid reasons. Whenever possible, therefore, they would arrange to postpone the discharge date.

Today, doctors are just as sympathetic to patients' need for recuperation time, but their ability to grant extended stays has been dramatically curtailed. The length of a patient's stay is not up to doctors anymore, but determined by an insurance-driven bureaucracy. As discussed in Chapter 5, "Dollars and Sense," strict DRG (Diagnosis-Related Groupings) guidelines assign fixed periods of stay for particular diagnoses and procedures. Hospitals earn money when patients are discharged quickly, and lose money if they linger. New hospital bureaucracies have mushroomed just to accelerate patients out of the hospital.

CONVALESCENCE AT HOME

Although most people leave the hospital healthier than when they arrived, they don't always actually feel better. Frequently, the treatment has been painful (e.g., surgery), or has even made them feel ill (chemotherapy). While both of these therapies are beneficial in the long run, they can weaken you in the short term. As a result, it is not unusual to leave the hospital not feeling 100 percent well. There will have to be a period of recuperation at home, sometimes even requiring skilled nursing care in the home.

Convalescence is a time to regain strength and readjust to normal life. How long this will take depends on your illness; your basic level of health; the support and help you have from family, friends, or home-care workers; and also your will to get better. Be patient! Returning to normal can take time.

Tips for a Smooth Convalescence

Discuss home-care plans with the social worker and nursing staff prior to discharge. Together, they can advise on the preparation of a safe environment for you to go home to. For example, you may require a hospital bed in your living room on the first floor if you can't climb stairs; a portable commode by the side of the bed if you can't walk; a chair in the bathtub to help with washing; a special diet; and someone to stay home with you twenty-four hours a day.

Alert your doctor to any possible problems as soon as possible. It is beyond the scope of this book to outline all the possible problems that may occur after a hospitalized patient has returned home. However, one of these three common, but serious problems should occasion a call to your doctor:

1. Excessive bleeding from anywhere: the surgical wound, the bowels, in the urine, or even from the gums.
2. High fever; any fever over 101-degrees Fahrenheit should at least be discussed with your doctor, unless you have been previously told to expect it.
3. Confusion; if this is a new problem, bring it to your physician's attention immediately.

Don't try to rush your recovery. It's understandable to chafe at the recuperation process, and natural to want to return as quickly as possible to your prehospital activities. But if you push yourself too soon, you may deprive yourself of the rest you need, and only succeed in *prolonging* your recuperation time.

Let your family and friends help you. Some people are better than others at accepting assistance from others. This is especially true if you tend to be a "can-do, take-care-of-things" type of person. Chances are you are more comfortable running ten errands for somebody else than in asking someone to run a single errand for you. Allow yourself to extend to others the gratifying experience of being helpers themselves. And remember: The more you rest now, the sooner you'll be back on your feet, and back in charge!

Arrange—or have someone arrange—for child care, meals, and perhaps a cleaning service. When you're healthy, whipping up a simple omelet takes five minutes. But when you're struggling to stand by the stove without hunching over from the pain of your incision, basic cooking can feel like an endurance test. Even for just a few days, try to get a break from the kitchen if possible.

If you have children, you probably won't want a complete break from them, but having someone take them to the park every afternoon so you can have some uninterrupted quiet can be a godsend. Explain to your children that it will be a while before you can play basketball in the driveway, or even make instant pudding, but that now is a good time for quiet activities such as reading or watching videos together or playing board games or cards.

HOME-CARE SERVICES

At the same time that insurance companies have tried to shorten hospital stays, they have also discovered that treatment at home is cheaper than hospital care. Insurers cover more extensive home-care options than ever before. Home-care services are provided through the interaction of the social worker, the floor nurses, the visting nurse service, and the department of home care, which coordinates all this activity. For example, let's follow George Fernandez, a seventy-eight-year-old man admitted to the neurology service with a major stroke. He is unable to speak or to move his right side when he first arrives at the hospital at ten o'clock one night. He is stabilized medically overnight, and the next morning, the nursing staff alerts the social worker assigned to the floor that Mr. Fernandez has been admitted. Ms. Brown, the social worker, comes to meet Mr. Fernandez and finds that although he can now speak, he still is unable to walk. She ascertains that he lives with his wife in a private home in Queens, New York, and that he is retired. He has Blue Cross/Blue Shield Medicare insurance coverage and a reasonable pension plan.

Ms. Brown writes in the chart that she feels that Mr. Fernandez will need some long-term discharge planning to include occupational and physical therapy to get him on his feet again; a cane and/or walker for ambulation; a temporary hospital bed if he cannot walk upstairs to his bedroom; and perhaps visiting nurse services at home if he is discharged on medications that need to be monitored. Ms. Brown has worked with many other patients with Mr. Fernandez's condition, and her experience alerts her to what he will probably need.

Ms. Brown speaks to the attending physician, then the nursing staff, then asks Mr. Fernandez's family to come and talk with her at the hospital. She explains what she has been doing and asks Mrs. Fernandez what the family's resources are, and whether she feels that she can ultimately care for Mr. Fernandez at home, depending on his level of recovery.

The dialogue between the patient's family and the social worker continues throughout the hospitalization as preparations are made for discharge. The ultimate needs will only become clear at the end of the hospitalization. How it is all ultimately arranged depends on a myriad of factors, including the patient's clinical state, family funds, and the number of children and their ability and willingness to help.

Among the most common home care services are:

Nursing care. Most insurance companies and Medicaid plans provide for visiting nurse services. Nurses make brief home visits to evaluate a patient's health problems; supervise care of long-term indwelling intravenous lines; change surgical dressings; check blood pressure; monitor medication use; and care for chronic bedsores. Frequently, they train patients' relatives in these and other tasks, and monitor their ability to safely provide care.

Nurses who care for patients with infectious diseases such as AIDS (acquired immunodeficiency syndrome), must also alert patients and their families to "universal precautions," protective ways to cope with blood and waste products to ensure that infection is not spread. Needles, gauze pads, sheets, towels, bloody bandages, and other items that may contain infected body fluids must be disposed of safely.

Home health aides. These are not nurses, but rather individuals trained to work with debilitated patients. Home health aides work up to twenty-four hours a day. They generally provide bed and bath care, and assist with aspects of daily living such as getting dressed, getting around, shopping for groceries, preparing meals, doing light house-cleaning and laundry. Medicaid will pay 100 percent of the cost of these services, even twenty-four-hour care, seven days a week. Medicare, however, only grants payment for four hours a day, no more than five days a week. As a consequence, enfeebled elderly patients frequently try to divest themselves of their assets in order to qualify for Medicaid and avail themselves of its benefits. HMOs (Health Maintenance Organizations—see Chapter 5, "Dollars and Sense") are quite strict about paying for these services, and must approve any home health aide visit.

Durable medical equipment. Many discharged patients require a variety of equipment to help them through the day. Crutches, wheelchairs, walkers, hospital beds, portable commodes, and other equipment can be rented, on a temporary or permanent basis, through the hospital's home-care department, delivered to your home with twenty-four hours' notice, and billed directly to your insurer, which generally pays the lion's share of the cost.

Occupational and physical therapy. These services, analogous to those provided in the hospital, are available for short periods of time at home. They must be ordered by your physician, and can be continued as long as the therapist believes they are necessary and helpful.

Home intravenous therapy. Subacute bacterial endocarditis is a bacterial infection of a heart valve that requires six weeks of intravenous antibiotics. Until a few years ago, a patient needed to spend the entire time as an inpatient. By the third week, most such patients felt well, and over the next three weeks, felt bored and frustrated by their hospital confinement. Today, a long-term intravenous line for the intermittent administration of antibiotics can be placed in the hospital and cared for at home by the patient, family members, and a nurse who comes in periodically. This saves thousands of dollars for insurance companies and frees patients to finish their treatment in the more convivial environment of their home. An entire industry has developed to administer these home intravenous programs, which also include chemotherapy for cancer, and hyperalimentation (intensive intravenous nourishment) for patients with trouble absorbing food through their gastrointestinal tract.

Glossary of Equipment

BEDPAN Triangular shallow pan made of metal or plastic, used by people who cannot get out of bed for bowel movements and urination.

BIOPSY NEEDLE Large needle which, after administration of local anesthesia, is passed through a person's skin in order to get a piece of tissue from a lump or tumor. The tissue is analyzed by a pathologist to determine if the lump or tumor is malignant or benign.

BLOW BOTTLE Device used by a patient to help keep lungs clear following surgery. (See *inspirometer.*)

CANE Walking stick a person holds in one hand to help maintain balance while walking, or to partially reduce the weight placed on an injured leg.

COMPRESSION STOCKINGS Leg coverings used to help keep the blood in the veins flowing back to the heart.

COOLING BLANKET Cover used to lower a patient's body temperature; often used when a patient has a high fever or during specialized types of anesthesia.

CRASH CART Portable chest with drawers for storage of drugs and lines used during CPR (cardiopulmonary resuscitation).

CRUTCHES   Supporting devices made of wooden or metal that are used as a walking aid. Crutches fit under the armpit and extend to the ground, and are usually used in pairs.

CYSTOSCOPE   Miniature fiber-optic device or television camera that enables a urologist to look inside a patient's bladder for tumors, stones, polyps, etc.

DEFIBRILLATOR   Life-saving instrument that uses an electrical charge or shock to restore the normal rhythm to the heart after a heart attack.

ECHOCARDIOGRAM   Study of the heart, its valves, and the motion of its walls using sound waves.

ELECTROCARDIOGRAM   Study of the electrical activity of the heart that checks the rhythm of the heart and can determine whether the heart has been damaged by a heart attack either in the past or presently.

ENDOSCOPE   Rigid or flexible instrument with a miniaturized light source and camera that enables a physician to see inside various areas of the body.

ENDOTRACHEAL TUBE   Anesthesia device placed through the mouth or the nose through the larynx and into the patient's trachea to help control respiration and protect the airway from aspiration of food and liquids while the patient is on a respirator or during anesthesia.

FORCEPS   Surgical instrument used for gently grasping tissue; obstetrical forceps are used to help deliver a baby.

GURNEY   Stretcher with wheels.

INSPIROMETER   Inhalation device used by patients to help keep lungs clear after surgery; in many hospitals, it replaces the blow bottle.

LARYNGOSCOPE   Lighted metal instrument through which an anesthesiologist views the vocal cords during insertion of an endotracheal tube.

LASER   (Acronym for light amplification by stimulated emission of radiation.) Form of high-energy light of a set wavelength that is used to destroy tumors, make incisions, and coagulate or seal blood vessels.

OPHTHALMOSCOPE   Lighted instrument through which a physician can look inside the eye and examine the back of the eyeball (the retina).

OSCILLOSCOPE   Small television monitor that displays an ongoing record of a wave form that may represent the electrical activity of the heart, the brain, or the changes in pressures in a blood vessel.

OTOSCOPE   Lighted instrument used to examine the outer parts of the ear and the eardrum.

PADDLES   The two ends of the defibrillator that are placed against the patient's chest when shock is used during cardiopulmonary resuscitation.

PULSE OXIMETER   Monitor that measures the amount of oxygen in the blood (oxygen saturation).

PUMP   Machine that pushes fluid at a constant rate through lines.

RESPIRATOR   Machine that breathes for a patient; not to be confused with the old type of iron lungs.

RETRACTOR   Surgical instrument used to hold a wound open or to shift the contents of a wound to the side during surgery to improve surgeons' view of the operating site.

SCALPEL   Surgical instrument used for making incisions and cutting tissue.

SCANNER   Machine that passes some sort of recording device over a part of the body or the whole body.

SPHYGMOMANOMETER   Instrument used to measure blood pressure.

STETHOSCOPE   Instrument used to listen to the sounds of the heart, lungs, and abdomen.

STRETCHER   Mobile bed used to transport patients.

SYRINGE   Narrow, hollow vial with an end for attaching a needle; used to carry fluids for injection or to draw off blood or other body fluids.

THERMOMETER   Instrument for measuring body temperature.

VENTILATOR   See *respirator*.

WALKER   Physical therapy aid to help a person walk.

X RAY   Study of the inside of the body recorded on a film similar to that used for photographs.

GLOSSARY OF PROCEDURES

AMYLASE TEST   Blood test to measure the levels of amylase, an enzyme from the pancreas. The higher the level of the serum amylase, the more likely that there is an injury, inflammation, infection, or other disease process (e.g., pancreatitis) involving the pancreas.

ANGIOGRAM   Invasive study of the blood vessels and the heart. A line is inserted in an artery in the arm or groin, which is then threaded through to the area to be studied, using X rays as a guide. Dye is then injected into the artery and X rays are taken of the area. Note: Some dyes have iodine, so patients allergic to iodine should inform their doctor.

ANGIOPLASTY   Invasive procedure using an inflatable balloon to correct a narrowing of a blood vessel. Usually performed on a blood vessel to the heart or to one of the legs when decreased diameter has reduced blood flow to these structures, causing angina (chest pain) or claudication (pain in the calves when walking).

APPENDECTOMY   Surgical removal of the appendix, a small vestigial outpouching of the intestine.

ARTHROSCOPY   Invasive orthopaedic procedure for treatment of injuries to the knee, shoulder, or other joints via endoscopy. The injuries seen may be secondary to trauma such as skiing accidents, aging, or arthritis. (See *endoscopy*.)

BARIUM ENEMA   X-ray study of the large intestine using barium, a type of dye; done to identify such problems as polyps, diverticuli, and tumors. After the intestine is cleaned out with enemas or laxatives, the barium is introduced into the intestine in the form of an enema. This highlights the area so that it shows up more clearly on an X ray.

BILATERAL SALPINGO-OOPHORECTOMY   Surgical removal of ovaries and fallopian tubes; commonly performed in conjunction with a hysterectomy.

BIOPSY   Surgical removal of a portion of tissue to be examined by a pathologist. The tissue is removed either by cutting with a scalpel or by sticking a large hollow needle into the tissue and studying the core of tissue left in the needle when it is withdrawn.

BLOOD TEST   Extraction of blood from an artery or vein for analysis.

BLOOD UREA NITROGEN (BUN)   Blood test to measure kidney function; usually performed in conjunction with a creatinine test. An elevated BUN result may indicate kidney problems, and may also indicate dehydration.

BONE SCAN   Study using injected radioactive dye to look for fractures, tumors, or infection in bone. Done by radiologist or a physician who specializes in nuclear medicine.

BREAST BIOPSY   Removal of a portion of tissue from a breast for examination by a pathologist; done with a needle or after making an incision with a scalpel.

BRONCHOSCOPY   Procedure for examining the trachea and bronchi of the lungs. Done by passing a flexible camera and light between the vocal cords and down into the trachea. Through direct visualization, the bronchoscopist can biopsy tumors, take cultures and washings, and visualize any pathology.

CANNULATE   Placement of a tube or wire into a hollow structure, commonly to drain a fluid or to inject a dye.

CARCINOEMBRYONIC ANTIGEN (CEA)   Enzyme measured in the blood. High or rising levels may indicate cancer.

CARDIAC CATHETERIZATION (ANGIOGRAM OF THE HEART)   Invasive radiological procedure using dye to study the heart's anatomy, motion, and blood vessels. A line is inserted into the skin and is passed through into an artery in the arm or the leg, then threaded under fluoroscopic (X-ray) guidance into the aorta and then into one of the arteries going directly to the heart.

CARDIAC VALVE REPLACEMENT   Surgical replacement of a damaged heart valve (usually the aortic or mitral valve) with an artificial (prosthetic) valve or one taken from a pig (porcine valve).

CASTING   Making a cast, a plaster, or fiberglass shell used to hold an extremity immobile in a precise position. Most commonly used to stabilize bone fractures, tendons, or muscles and joints.

CATARACT   Growth in the lens of the eye that interferes with vision; most commonly occurs in older adults.

CAT SCAN   Also known as a CT scan or computerized tomography. Thin bands of X rays are used to make detailed composite pictures of cross sections of the body. The pictures are then assembled and re-formatted by computer so that the part of the body that is being studied can be viewed from several angles and directions.

CHEST TUBE   Line inserted into the space around the lungs, to remove fluids and gases and to keep the lungs fully expanded. This procedure is usually necessary after most thoracic and cardiac surgery, or after trauma or the spontaneous collapse of the lung (pneumothorax).

CHEST X RAY   X-ray study of the heart and the lungs to study function and to detect infection and tumors. Required for all patients over the age of forty who are undergoing surgery.

CHOLECYSTECTOMY   Surgical removal of the gallbladder.

COLECTOMY   Surgical removal of part or all of the intestine, usually due to diverticulosis or colon tumors.

COLONOSCOPY   Internal examination of the intestines using a flexible colonoscope. This instrument, which is inserted through the rectum, has a small television camera and light source for viewing the rectum and the colon to examine for polyps, tumors, diverticuli, etc.

COLOSTOMY (STOMA)   Surgically created opening into the intestine, which takes over the function of the bowel. The feces collects in a colostomy bag, which hangs from the site of the incision. Colostomy is often done as a temporary measure to allow the bowel to heal after infection or surgery; after this healing process, the colostomy is surgically closed.

COLPOSCOPY   Examination of the cervix and uterus.

COMPLETE BLOOD COUNT (CBC)   Blood test to measure hemoglobin, hematocrit, and the number of red blood cells, white blood cells (of various types), and platelets. Aids diagnosis of such conditions as anemia (hemoglobin and hematocrit are too low), leukemia (excessive production of white blood cells), and thrombocytopenia (excessive bleeding caused by inadequate production of platelets).

CORONARY ARTERY BYPASS GRAFTING (CABG)   (The acronym is pronounced *cabbage.*) Surgical correction of a blockage in the arteries to the heart. There are three main arteries to the heart from the aorta: the left, the right, and the circumflex. A patient may require one to five bypass grafts (usually veins taken from the leg) to correct the main blockages.

CRANIOTOMY   Neurosurgical opening of the cranium or skull to remove a tumor, correct bleeding, or relieve pressure (e.g., hydrocephalus).

CREATININE   Blood test to measure kidney function; usually performed in conjunction with the BUN (blood urea). A physician may request that the patient collect urine for twenty-four hours to measure the creatinine clearance.

CRYOSURGERY   Destruction of tissue using nitrogen.

CURETTAGE   Scraping of tissue for debridement, destruction, or biopsy. Performed with a curette, an instrument consisting of a long metal handle attached to a small round scoop with sharp edges for cutting.

CYSTOSCOPY   Procedure during which a urologist uses a cystoscope to look inside the bladder for tumors and other problems. The cystoscope consists of a small camera, light source, and irrigation tube, which is passed through the urethra into the bladder.

DEBRIDEMENT   Surgical removal of diseased, infected, or dead tissue, often for patients burned in fires, injured in car accidents, or afflicted with bed sores (pressure sores).

DIALYSIS   Cleansing of the blood to remove impurities that have accumulated because of kidney failure or malfunction. *Hemodialysis*, required by patients on long-term dialysis, is the direct removal from a patient's bloodstream of impurities that have collected in the blood. *Peritoneal dialysis* is the irrigating out of the patient's abdominal cavity with a cleansing fluid; generally done when dialysis is believed to be temporary (as opposed to a life-long treatment).

DILATATION AND CURETTAGE (D & C)   Dilatation is the widening of the opening of the cervix (the end of the uterus at the deepest part of the vagina) in order for the gynecologist to gain access to the uterus for curettage, during which the lining is scraped. Frequently done to treat women with excessive vaginal bleeding or after miscarriage. (See *curettage*.)

DRAIN   Line or device left in place to allow fluids to be eliminated from the body, frequently after surgery. Also refers to the removal of fluids—usually blood, serum, or pus—that may have collected secondary to infection or after trauma.

ECHOCARDIOGRAM   Study of the heart's anatomy, valve function, and motion using sound waves; can help diagnose valve abnormalities such as mitral valve prolapse (MVP).

ELECTROCARDIOGRAM (ECG OR EKG)   Study of the electrical activity of the heart to determine abnormal rhythm, other heart diseases, and whether a patient has ever had a heart attack. Performed by placing twelve electrodes (leads) on the patient, one attached to each arm and leg and the remainder placed across the chest.

ELECTROENCEPHALOGRAM (EEG)   Study of the electrical activity (brain-wave pattern) of the brain; done by attaching many electrodes to the patient's scalp. Used to help diagnose epilepsy. In many states, the absence of brain waves must be documented on an EEG in order to declare a patient brain-dead.

ELECTROLYTES   Sodium, potassium, and carbon dioxide are all electrolytes, substances in the blood which help regulate electrical activity in the body. Changes in the levels of these electrolytes are affected by many conditions and drugs. For example, people who take large amounts of diuretics can dangerously reduce the serum level of their potassium. A person with an adrenal tumor may have a markedly altered serum sodium. An electrolyte test is done to determine the levels of these substances in the blood.

ELECTROMYELOGRAM (EMG)   Study of the electrical activity of muscle, done to detect problems with the peripheral nerves, such as carpal tunnel syndrome.

ENDARTERECTOMY   Invasive procedure for the removal of disease inside a blood vessel. Carotid endarterectomy, performed by a neurosurgeon or vascular surgeon, involves the removal of a blockage in the carotid arteries that provide blood to the brain.

ENDOSCOPY   Study of the inside of the body via a miniaturized television camera. Procedures that can be performed endoscopically include appendectomy, colectomy, face lifts, gallbladder removal, hysterectomy, and tummy tucks.

EXCISION   Removal of tissue or a tumor which is then sent to a pathologist for study.

EXERCISE STRESS TEST   Study of the heart during exercise to determine if there is any disease in vessels that supply blood to the heart. While the patient runs on a treadmill or rides a reclining bicycle, the ECG is continuously monitored. Often done by a cardiologist in conjunction with a physician specializing in nuclear medicine in order to obtain pictures of the motion of the heart.

FLAT PLATE   X ray, usually of the abdomen; used to determine such problems as bowel obstruction or perforation.

FOLEY CATHETER   Tube passed through the urethra into the bladder which drains the urine from the bladder. Done during some long surgeries, and in patients whose enlarged prostates obstruct urination. The foley catheter also is used to assess how a patient's cardiac and renal systems are performing, as it provides a direct measurement of urine production. This is especially helpful for patients in the ICU.

GASTRECTOMY   Surgical removal of all or part of the stomach. Most commonly done for ulcer or tumors, it is occasionally done on morbidly obese patients to promote weight loss.

GLUCOSE   Blood sugar; glucose test is a simple blood test used to diagnose *diabetes* (abnormal ability to control the levels of blood sugar, which is normally controlled by insulin, a hormone produced by the pancreas) and *hypoglycemia* (abnormally low blood sugar).

GUAIAC   Method of detecting the presence of blood, usually in the stool. A physician places a sample of the patient's stool on a special card that has been treated with guaiac liquid. The card will turn a particular color in the presence of blood—an indication that a patient may have slow bleeding ulcers, polyps, or colon cancer.

HEMATOCRIT   The proportion of the blood that is composed of red blood cells. (See *complete blood count.*)

HEMOGLOBIN   The part of the red blood cell to which oxygen attaches in the lungs, so that it can be transported throughout the body. (See *complete blood count.*)

HERNIORRHAPHY   Surgical repair of a hernia. The most common type of hernia is an inguinal (groin) hernia. Hernias that occur after surgery are known as incisional hernias.

INCISION AND DRAINAGE (I & D)   Procedure in which a small incision or opening is made to drain or remove fluid, usually infected (pus). Cures infection, relieves discomfort, and helps diagnose the bacteria causing the infection.

INTRAVENOUS (IV) LINES   Tubes that allow fluids, such as blood or saline (salt) solution, to enter the veins; used, for example, for patients in surgery; in an intensive care unit; or when receiving chemotherapy. Common types of intravenous fluids are normal saline, Ringer's lactate, and D5W (5 percent glucose in water), and albumiso.

INTRAVENOUS PYELOGRAM (IVP)   X-ray study of the kidneys, ureters, and bladder that use dye. The dye is injected directly into the patient's blood. Patients who are allergic to dyes, or to iodine, should inform the radiologist or urologist before the procedure.

INTUBATION   Insertion of an endotracheal tube into a patient's trachea. Controls a patient's respiration during general anesthesia, or in an intensive care unit for critically ill patients. The outer end of the endotracheal tube is attached to a respirator that automatically breathes for the patient, or to an "ambu bag," which must be squeezed by the doctor, nurse, or other health care professional in order to make it breathe for the patient.

LAMINECTOMY   Surgery on the back performed by a neurosurgeon, or by an orthopaedic surgeon, to relieve severe back pain or pain that radiates down the legs from a slipped disc.

LAPAROSCOPY   Surgical procedure where a miniaturized television camera is used to look inside the abdomen. Done for diagnostic or therapeutic reasons. For example, a gynecologist may laparoscopically look at a tumor of the ovary and biopsy a portion of it for diagnosis or remove it for definitive treatment.

LAPAROTOMY   Surgical opening of the abdomen; refers to any open abdominal procedure, such as cholecystectomy, colectomy, or hysterectomy.

LARYNGOSCOPY   Surgical procedure for visual study of the larynx, e.g., to identify polyps or nodules. Usually done under sedation or with a topical anesthetic.

LIVER FUNCTION TESTS   Blood tests to measure the function of the liver by measuring specific enzymes (alk. phos., LDH, SGOT, SGPT, etc.). These enzymes are elevated in such infectious disorders as hepatitis and mononucleosis. Liver function tests are also abnormal in noninfectious disorders such as gallbladder disease.

LIVER SCAN   Study of the liver requiring the injection of a radioactive agent into the patient's blood. Used to find abnormalities in the liver, such as cysts or tumors that have metastasized to the liver.

LUMPECTOMY   Removal of a breast tumor or portion of the breast; not a total removal of the breast. Often combined with radiation therapy for treatment of breast cancers in patients who are not going to be treated with a mastectomy.

MAGNETIC RESONANCE IMAGING (MRI)   Noninvasive scan that gives detailed information about the anatomy and any abnormalities; performed by radiologists. Involves spending approximately one hour on a table inside a tight circular machine; some MRIs, however, are open, an experience that patients find less claustrophobic, but which may not produce results as reliable as those of closed machines.

MASTECTOMY, MODIFIED   Removal of the breast and the lymph nodes under the arm, but not the pectoralis muscle; treats carcinoma of the breast. Some patients also choose to undergo a breast reconstruction at the time of mastectomy.

MASTECTOMY, RADICAL   Removal of the breast, the pectoralis muscle, and the lymph nodes under the arm. Less commonly done today than twenty years ago, when it was the treatment of choice for breast cancer.

MASTECTOMY, SIMPLE   Removal of the breast without removing any lymph nodes from under the arm or removing the pectoralis muscle. Most commonly done for a malignant tumor of the breast; also performed prophylactically for patients with a strong family history of breast cancer or who have already been diagnosed with cancer in the other breast.

NEEDLE BIOPSY   Use of a needle to remove a portion of tissue for study by a pathologist.

NEPHRECTOMY   Surgical removal of a kidney, or a portion of a kidney.

OCCUPATIONAL THERAPY   Type of physical therapy concerned primarily with the functions of the hand; occupational therapists make complex splints, and other devices, to help patients regain use of their hand after surgery or trauma, and play a critical role in patient care in many burn centers.

OPEN REDUCTION INTERNAL FIXATION OF FRACTURES   Surgical treatment of a fracture. *Open* refers to the fact that an incision is made in the skin. *Internal* refers to metal plates, wires, and pins placed in or against the bone to stabilize it in its normal anatomic position so that it can heal.

PACEMAKER   Medical device placed by a cardiac surgeon that controls the heartbeat rate. The pacemaker is usually permanently placed under the skin over the upper part of the chest. A lead from the pacemaker is placed inside a vein and guided into the heart to monitor and stimulate the beating of the heart as necessary.

PACKING   Gauze placed inside a space in the body, e.g., to control bleeding following surgery, or as a daily dressing for treatment of an abscess cavity.

PAP SMEAR   Study of the cells of the cervix to determine whether there is a malignancy; a routine part of regular gynecological examinations. The cervix is gently scraped with a wooden stick, then the collected cells are spread out on a glass slide for study by a pathologist.

Researchers disagree about whether women should have a pap smear every year or every two years.

PARACENTESIS   Removal of a collection of fluid by inserting a needle through the skin; used for both diagnostic and therapeutic reasons. (See *thoracentesis.)*

PHYSICAL THERAPY OR PHYSIOTHERAPY   Therapy or treatment for joints, muscles, and tendons; prescribed by physiatrists and provided by physical and occupational therapists.

PLATELETS   Structure in blood that promotes clotting. Platelet levels that are too low (thrombocytopenia) can cause spontaneous bleeding or excessive bleeding during and after surgery. Levels that are too high (thrombocytosis) can cause spontaneous formation of clots inside a person's blood vessels and may lead to extensive tissue damage.

PROSTATE SPECIFIC ANTIGEN (PSA)   Blood test to detect the presence of prostate cancer; should probably be monitored routinely in all men over the age of forty-five or fifty.

RADIONUCLIDE   A radioactive substance absorbed in the body; used for diagnostic X-ray tests called nuclear medical scans.

SEDIMENTATION RATE (ESR)   Nonspecific blood test used to detect the presence or absence of infection or inflammation in the body. Used by doctors both as a diagnostic screening tool, and as a method to follow the resolution, or clinical course, of disease or infection.

SIGMOIDOSCOPY   Study of the lower part of the large intestine in which a hollow, rigid tube, or a flexible endoscope, is inserted in the rectum; important in the early detection of colon cancer.

SONOGRAM   Noninvasive radiological study of the inside of the body using sound waves. Often employed during pregnancy to follow and assess the development of the fetus.

SPINAL TAP   Insertion of a needle between two vertebrae, and into the space around the spinal cord, that removes a small portion of spinal fluid in order to detect infection—or diseases such as multiple sclerosis.

SPLINTING   Method of supporting the body in a prescribed position, using materials such as plaster, plastic, and metal. Splinting allows an injured muscle or joint to rest; to actively rehabilitate an injured tendon; or to immobilize an arm or leg immediately after surgery (e.g., after skin grafting) to allow for proper healing.

STAPEDECTOMY   Removal of a portion of the bones of the middle ear, usually to improve hearing in patients who have suffered hearing loss.

THALLIUM STRESS TEST   Nuclear-medicine test in which a radionuclide is used to visualize the activity of the heart during exercise. (See *exercise stress test*.)

THORACENTESIS   Insertion of a needle into the thorax or chest to remove fluid from around the lungs. Often used to detect cells of tumors. (See *paracentesis*.)

THYROID FUNCTION TESTS   Blood tests used to asses thyroid function. A patient whose thyroid is not producing enough thyroid hormone is treated with replacement hormones.

THYROID SCAN   Noninvasive use of a radionuclide to assess thyroid function, or to detect the presence of tumors. Performed by a nuclear physician or a radiologist.

TONSILLECTOMY   Surgical removal of the tonsils because of repeated, severe infection; one of the most common surgical procedures of childhood. Sometimes involves removal of the adenoids.

TOTAL ABDOMINAL HYSTERECTOMY   Removal of the uterus and cervix for treatment of malignancies and certain benign conditions such as fibroids.

TOTAL JOINT REPLACEMENT   Replacement of a joint with an artificial one, most commonly due to arthritis caused by trauma, aging, or rheumatoid disease. Most often involves the hip and the knee joints, although most joints, including elbow, wrist, and fingers, can be replaced.

TRANSURETHRAL PROSTATECTOMY   Removal of part of the prostate by operating directly through the urethra; treats benign prostatic hypertrophy (BPH), enlargement of the prostate. Performed when prostate becomes so enlarged that it obstructs the urethra and prevents urination.

ULTRASOUND   Use of sound waves to study anatomy and structure. (See *sonogram*.)

UPPER GI SERIES Noninvasive X-ray study of the esophagus, stomach, and small intestine using dye; patient must drink liquid barium prior to the procedure. Aids diagnosis of ulcers and tumors.

URINALYSIS Study of a urine sample for blood cells (red and white), bacteria, other cells, sugar, stones, and other tests. An important screening test in routine physical examinations and for patients who are undergoing surgery. A urinalysis can detect such problems as diabetes, kidney infection, and bladder tumors.

WASHINGS Irrigation of cells with fluid, usually saline solution, to collect cells for study by a pathologist for detection of infection or malignancy. Washings are often performed at the time of bronchoscopy to detect lung cancer.

WHITE BLOOD CELL (WBC) COUNT Test to determine the numbers of white cells in the blood; part of a complete blood count. These cells are used to fight infection and their number is usually fewer than ten thousand. Patients who are receiving chemotherapy have a reduced number of white blood cells (leukopenia) and, therefore, have a reduced ability to fight infection. Patients with an elevated WBC count (leukocytosis) may have an infection (WBC usually between ten and twenty thousand) or leukemia (very high WBC count). (See *complete blood count.*)

GLOSSARY OF COMMONLY
USED DRUGS

The following is a brief summary of the most commonly used drugs in a hospital. Not all the drugs in each class of drugs can be included because of space limitations, nor can all the effects and side effects be described. For a complete discussion of each drug's strengths, weaknesses, uses, contraindications and side effects, consult your physician or the *PDR (Physician's Desk Reference)*.

ACETOMINOPHEN (TYLENOL)   A non-aspirin pain reliever. Commonly used in hospitals for headaches and minor pains.

ADRIAMYCIN   An anticancer drug. Used extensively for breast cancer and many leukemias, it has many toxic side effects.

ADVIL   Nonsteroidal pain reliever used mainly for arthritis pains. May also be used for headaches, premenstrual syndrome, and injuries. Now sold over the counter.

ALEVE   Nonsteroidal pain reliever used mainly for arthritis pains. May also be used for headaches, premenstrual syndrome, and injuries. Sold over the counter.

ALLOPURINOL (XYLOPRIM)   A pill taken every day to prevent gout.

ALPHABLOCKERS   Antihypertensive drugs, now more commonly used to alleviate the symptoms of prostate enlargement in men. The best known is Hytrin.

AMINOPHYLLINE   An oral or intravenous medication for the treatment of the wheezing of asthma.

AMPHOTERICIN   An antifungal agent used intravenously. Has many severe side effects such as high fevers, and generally used in patients who are immune compromised because of cancer chemotherapy.

ANGIOTENSIN CONVERTING ENZYME INHIBITORS (ACE INHIBITORS)   Initially conceived of as antihypertensive medications, they are now also used for relief of congestive heart failure and in certain kidney problems. Best known are Vasotec and Capoten.

ANTIBIOTICS   Medications used to cure bacterial infections such as an abscess. They have no effect on viruses. Many different varieties are now tailored for specific germs and illnesses.

ANTICOAGULANT   A medication to inhibit blood clotting. Commonly known as blood thinners, but do not actually thin the blood in any way. Used in many forms (Coumadin, aspirin, Persantine) and for many different conditions. Do not totally stop clotting, only slow it down.

ASPIRIN   An anti-inflammatory agent and pain reliever. May also protect against heart attacks and strokes due to a mild anti-blood clotting effect.

AUGMENTIN   A penicillin-based antibiotic. Used mainly for ear and sinus infections.

AXID   Prevents the production of acid in the stomach. Used to cure ulcers and for severe heartburn. The original drug of this group is Tagamet.

BENADRYL   An antihistamine used to alleviate allergy symptoms of runny nose, teary eyes, itching, and sneezing. Causes drowsiness and is therefore also used as a sleeping aide.

BENZODIAZAPINE   A class of drugs used for anxiety disorders and sleep disturbances. May be habit forming. Subject to strict government control due to potential for abuse.

BETA BLOCKERS   A large group of drugs used for angina (chest pain), hypertension, heart rhythm abnormalities, tremor, and even stage fright. Best known are Inderal (propranolol) and Lopressor (metoprolol).

BETOPTIC   An eyedrop used in the treatment of glaucoma (elevated pressure in the eye).

CALCIUM CHANNEL BLOCKERS   A group of drugs with many different effects. Used for hypertension, angina, heart rhythm abnormalities. Best known are Cardizem and verapamil.

CAPOTEN (CAPTOPRIL)   An angiotensin-converting enzyme inhibitor. The first of this group of drugs used for the treatment of hypertension, congestive heart failure, and after heart attacks.

CARDIZEM   See *calcium channel blockers.*

CASCARA   A colonic irritant to prevent constipation.

CEPHALOSPORINS   A class of antibiotics. The original and best known is Keflex.

CHEMOTHERAPY   A drug regimen used in an attempt to cure or control cancer. Frequently used as a group of several medications given in a specific pattern for specific malignancies and individual patients.

CHLORAL HYDRATE   A sleep medication. May be habit forming.

COLACE   A prescription stool softener to prevent constipation.

COLCHICINE   A medication to prevent or control the pain of acute attacks of gout.

COMPAZINE   A drug to prevent nausea and vomiting.

COUMADIN   An anticoagulant. Must be carefully monitored lest it "thins" the blood excessively and provokes bleeding.

CYCLOSPORINE   A drug which suppresses the immune system. Used for treating lupus and other hyperimmune states and to prevent the rejection of transplanted organs.

CYTOXAN   Chemo (drug) therapy for cancer. Used to treat a variety of different malignancies, including breast cancer and lymphoma (cancer of the lymph glands).

DALMANE A benzodiazapine sleeping medication. Same class of drugs as Valium. May be habit forming.

DEMEROL A narcotic pain reliever. May be habit forming.

DIABETA A pill to lower blood sugar in diabetics. Used in conjunction with diet and weight loss in non-insulin-dependent diabetics.

DIGOXIN (LANOXIN, DIGITALIS) Derived from the plant foxglove two hundred years ago and still used for congestive heart failure and certain heart rhythm abnormalities.

DILANTIN An anti-epilepsy (seizure) drug.

DILAUDID A narcotic pain reliever.

DIURETICS Commonly called "water pills," because they stimulate urination. In reality, they cause the kidneys to excrete salt, and water goes along to dissolve the salt so it can be discharged in the urine. Most common are Lasix (furosemide) and hydrochlorthiazide (hydrodiuril).

DOPAMINE An intravenous drug used to raise the blood pressure in severely ill patients with low blood pressure. Also enhances kidney function and improves the pumping of the heart.

ELAVIL (AMYTRIPTILINE) An antidepressant. Also occasionally used to treat chronic pain and spasticity.

ERYTHROMYCIN See *antibiotics.*

ESTROGENS Female reproductive hormones. Produced naturally in the body until menopause; some post-menopausal women take synthetic estrogen replacement (ERT), which are taken orally. Also used in birth control pills.

FELDENE See *nonsteroidal.*

GO-LYTELY A laxative agent used to clean out the bowels. Usually given the night before a bowel procedure (such as a colonoscopy).

HALDOL An antipsychotic medication, frequently used in hospitals to quiet patients who are confused and combative.

HEPARIN An intravenous anticoagulant. Used to dissolve and prevent clots from forming.

HYDROCHLORTHIAZIDE   One of the earliest and most commonly used diuretics. The major side effect is loss of potassium in the urine, which can usually be corrected by increasing potassium in the diet by eating bananas.

HYTRIN   See *alphablockers.*

IMMODIUM   An over-the-counter medication to control diarrhea.

IMMURAN   A drug that suppresses the immune system. Used in transplant patients (heart, kidney, liver) to prevent rejection of the new organ.

INDERAL   The original beta blocker. Used in hypertension, angina, heart rhythm abnormalities, and even for stage fright.

INSULIN   An injected hormone used to control the level of blood sugar in people with diabetes, a disease in which the pancreas does not secrete enough insulin.

ISONIAZID (INH)   An antituberculosis medication.

KAOPECTATE   Liquid plant fiber used to combat diarrhea.

KEFLEX   See *antibiotics.*

LASIX   One of the most powerful diuretics.

LESCOL   A drug to lower elevated cholesterol levels.

LEVOPHED   A powerful cardiac stimulant used intravenously. Raises the blood pressure and helps the heart to pump more vigorously.

LIBRIUM   A benzodiazapine, antianxiety agent. The mildest of the group.

LOMOTIL   A prescription medication used to control diarrhea.

LOPRESSOR   See *beta blockers.*

MAALOX   An antacid used for heartburn and ulcers.

MAGNESIUM CITRATE   A colonic irritant that cleanses and helps empty the intestinal tract.

METHOTREXATE   An anticancer drug. See *chemotherapy.*

MEVACOR   A drug to lower elevated cholesterol levels.

MICRONASE   See *oral hypoglycemics.*

MILK OF MAGNESIA   A milky liquid used to induce bowel movements and prevent constipation.

MINOXYDIL (ROGAINE)   A cream or liquid rubbed into the scalp to promote hair growth. Initially developed as an antihypertensive, it was found to cause excessive hair growth.

MORPHINE   A narcotic pain reliever. Also used for acute heart failure.

MOTRIN   See *nonsteroidal.*

MYLANTA   An antacid used for heartburn and ulcers.

NAPROSYN   See *nonsteroidal.*

NAVANE   An antipsychotic medication.

NITROGLYCERIN   The oldest known medication for angina (chest/heart pain). Slipped under the tongue and allowed to dissolve, or used as a spray, it can halt an angina attack in minutes. Also available in longer acting preparations (nitrates, Nitrostat, Isordil).

NONSTEROIDAL ANTIINFLAMMATORY DRUGS (NSAID)   Pain relievers mainly used for arthritis pains. May also be used for headaches, premenstrual syndrome, and injuries. Now many are sold over the counter (Advil, Motrin, Aleve).

ORAL HYPOGLYCEMICS   Pills used to lower the level of blood sugar in diabetes.

PAXIL   An antidepressant.

PENICILLIN   See *antibiotics.*

PHENOBARBITOL   A barbiturate antianxiety drug. Also used to prevent seizures associated with epilepsy.

PRAVACHOL   A drug to lower elevated cholesterol levels.

PREDNISONE   The most commonly used oral steroid. (See *steroids.*)

PRILOSEC   A special antacid pill used for irritation in the esophagus.

PROCARDIA   See *calcium channel blockers.*

PRONESTYL   An antiarrhythmic used for heart rhythm abnormalities.

PROPULSID   Enhances the propulsion of food in the gastrointestinal tract.

PROZAC   An antidepressant.

QUINIDINE   An antiarrhythmic drug used for heart rhythm abnormalities.

RELAFEN   See *nonsteroidal.*

RETIN-A   An acne medication.

RIFAMPIN   An antituberculosis medication, occasionally also used as an antibiotic.

SINEMET   A pill to control the symptoms of Parkinson's disease (e.g., excessive tremors).

STEROIDS   Short form for corticosteroids. Hormones produced in the body by the adrenal glands. As medications, used to relieve inflammation and to treat cancer, asthma, and arthritis. Most commonly used is prednisone.

STREPTOKINASE   A clot-buster used for heart attacks and strokes. Works best in the first four hours after the onset of symptoms.

SUDAFED (PSEUDOEPHEDRINE)   A decongestant used for colds and allergies to reduce congestion in the ears and nose.

SYNTHROID   Synthetic thyroid hormone. Replaces thyroid hormone for people whose own thyroid gland produces insufficient quantities; also used to treat goiters (enlarged thyroid glands).

TAGAMET   A drug used to prevent the production of acid in the stomach. Used to cure ulcers and for severe heartburn.

TENORMIN   See *beta blockers.*

TETRACYCLINE   See *antibiotics.*

THEODUR   A drug to help prevent and cure the wheezing of asthma attacks.

THORAZINE   An antipsychotic drug which has also been used to control hiccups.

TIMOPTIC   An eyedrop used for the treatment of glaucoma.

TOFRANIL   An antidepressant.

TPA (TISSUE PLASMINOGEN ACTIVATOR, "CLOT-BUSTER")   An intravenous medication used to rapidly dissolve clots in patients with acute heart attacks. Works best within four hours of the onset of the heart attack.

TYLENOL   A pain reliever and anti-fever medication. Contains no aspirin.

URSODEOXYCHOLINE   A pill that dissolves some types (cholesterol) of gallstones, sometimes eliminating the need for gallbladder surgery.

VALIUM   A benzodiazapine antianxiety medication. One of the most prescribed drugs in the United States.

VANCOMYCIN   An intravenous antibiotic.

VASOTEC   See *angiotensin converting enzyme inhibitors.*

VENTOLIN   A spray or pill used to treat asthma.

VERAPAMIL   See *calcium channel blockers.*

VERSED   An anesthetic. Puts patients to sleep rapidly.

WELBUTRIN   An antidepressant.

ZANTAC   A drug to prevent the production of acid in the stomach, used to prevent and cure ulcers.

ZOCOR   A drug to lower elevated cholesterol levels.

ZOLOFT   An antidepressant.

INDEX

362.11   Tyberg, Theodore.
T
          Surviving your
            hospitalization.

$23.00

	DATE		

1/4/96

BAKER & TAYLOR